"For anyone beginning the second half of life, *The Power Years* will psych you up for the great adventure ahead."

　　　　　—Po Bronson, author of *What Should I Do With My Life?*

"In the field of 'middlescence,' as he calls it, Ken Dychtwald is the master. I count on his brilliance, his pioneering ideas, his courage, and his optimism and we would all be poorer without him. I recommend *The Power Years* without reservation. It is a must read."

　　　　　—Richard N. Bolles, author of *What Color Is Your Parachute?*

"I have been learning from Ken Dychtwald for years and am convinced that he is today's most original thinker on this important subject."

　　　　　—President Jimmy Carter

"While powerful and complex currents of demographic change are sweeping the globe, little has been said about what the post–World War II generation wants from later life. In *The Power Years*, Dychtwald and Kadlec provide a well-informed and optimistic roadmap for how this new chapter of life need not be a period of retreat and decline, but instead holds the potential for becoming a time of renewal and personal reinvention."

　　　　　—Sir John Bond, Chairman of HSBC Holdings plc

"Dychtwald sees the creation of a whole new multi-decade stage of life . . . a period that offers rich opportunities for reinvention and exploration. . . . Dychtwald is the perfect spokesman for the coming change."

　　　　　—*Fortune* magazine

"If you want to make your future years the best years ever—to feel ageless and experience a dynamic, purposeful, joyful, and full life—read *The Power Years*."

—Mark Victor Hansen, co-creator of the #1 *New York Times* bestselling *Chicken Soup for the Soul* series and coauthor of *The One Minute Millionaire*

"Ken Dychtwald and Daniel J. Kadlec have written a fantastic book filled with compelling data and anecdotes that show that the so-called declining years are anything but. *The Power Years* helped rid me of much of my worry about what lies ahead and gave me specific, solid ideas for how to make the next 50 years top the first 50 for financial success, career satisfaction, and overall fun."

—James J. Cramer, author of *Jim Cramer's Real Money: Sane Investing in an Insane World,* CNBC commentator, and cofounder of *TheStreet.com*

The Power Years

A User's Guide to
the Rest of Your Life

Ken Dychtwald, Ph.D.
and
Daniel J. Kadlec

WILEY

John Wiley & Sons, Inc.

Published by John Wiley & Sons, Inc., Hoboken, New Jersey
Published simultaneously in Canada

Design and composition by Navta Associates, Inc.

For general information about our other products and services, please contact our Customer Care Department within the United States at (800) 762-2974, outside the United States at (317) 572-3993 or fax (317) 572-4002.

Wiley also publishes its books in a variety of electronic formats. Some content that appears in print may not be available in electronic books. For more information about Wiley products, visit our web site at www.wiley.com.

Library of Congress Cataloging-in-Publication Data:

Dychtwald, Ken, date.
  The power years : a user's guide to the rest of your life / Ken Dychtwald, and Daniel J. Kadlec.
      p. cm.
  Includes bibliographical references and index.
  ISBN-13 978-0-471-67494-8 (cloth)
  ISBN-10 0-471-67494-X (cloth)
  1. Life skills.   I. Kadlec, Daniel J.   II. Title.
  HQ2037.D93 2005
  646.7'0084'4—dc22

                                                            2005007115

Printed in the United States of America

10 9 8 7 6 5 4 3 2 1

For Pearl and Seymour Dychtwald,
who have breathed life, spirit, and hope
into every second of my life

—Ken Dychtwald

For my dear love, Kim, and our
joyful children, Lexie, Kyle, and
Danielle, who inspire me daily

—Daniel J. Kadlec

Contents

Acknowledgments

In writing this book we have drawn from many sources in addition to incorporating our own studies and many interviews. Throughout the text and in notes at the end we give credit where it's due. But we owe special thanks to many folks who helped us shape our thoughts and values, sometimes over decades, and to those who helped us gather the information we needed and present it in this final form. Both authors would like to recognize Owen Laster and Tom Miller, our wonderful agent and gifted editor, who empowered us to bring this special book to life. We also recognize Tom Franco, the communications wizard most responsible for bringing us together. We further offer these individual acknowledgments.

From Ken:
I would like to thank the following very special people for their enormous contributions to my life and work:

Maddy Kent Dychtwald, my true soulmate, for your unrivaled radiance and for being my dream come true. Casey Dychtwald for your fantastic appetite for self-empowerment. Zak

Dychtwald for your kindhearted and ancient wisdom. Alan Dychtwald for your generosity of spirit and for cheering me on every day of my life.

Sally and Ray Fusco, Richard, Linda, David, and Joel Kent for nourishing us Kent-Dychtwalds with respect and affection. Elyse Pellman for your mastery of the positive. Robyn Hamilton for your extraordinary intelligence and kindness. David Baxter for your shining and complex brilliance. My dearest friends, Kenny and Sandie Dorman, Jayme and Gayle Canton, Danny and Nancy Katz, Bill and Jill Burkart, Elyse and Stuart Pellman, Chip Baird and Brent Knudsen—for your empathy, complexity, sympathy, proximity, and adversity (what are friends for?).

Bob Morison, Tammy Erickson, Ron Christman, Bruce Clark, Mark Goldstein, Bart Penfold, Diane Barde, Stacy Nelson, Erin Pritchett, Luke Van Meter, Matt Mucklo, Neil Steinberg, Aaron Vance, Catherine Fredman, Brandon Buttrick, Andy Nussbaum, Nancy Lunney, Gordon Wheeler, Michael Murphy, George Leonard, Nancy Worcester, Serena D'arcy Fisher, Ann Downing, Stu Weinstein, Lucia Rose Horan, Don and Catherine Mankin, Frank and Claire Wuest, Bill and Mary Lou Newman— what a fabulous cast of characters!

From Dan:
This book—indeed, my career as a writer—would not be possible without the unflinching support of my insightful and brilliant wife, Kim, who has more good ideas in an hour than most people have in a lifetime. I also acknowledge the invaluable contributions of my sparkling children: Lexie, whose grit and unbowed sense of discovery keep me sharp; Kyle, whose generosity, kindness, and humor constantly remind me of what matters most in life; and Danielle, whose pluck, effervescent personality and glowing smile are the energy field that sustains me. Thank you all for cheerfully suffering my consistent requests to "please find

something else to do tonight because Dad needs the computer." Note to family: You may have the keyboard back.

I also recognize my father, Edwin, who has forever been a perfect role model, and my mother, Audrey, for her steady love.

Special thanks go to my editors at *Time* magazine, most notably Jim Kelly and Steve Koepp, who graciously allowed me a leave of absence for this project. I also recognize the superb *Time* research staff, which is so adept at filling in missing pieces: Jim Oberman, Kathleen Dowling, Suzy Im, Susan Kramer, Charlie Lampach, and Angela Thornton. Finally, some of the material in this book previously appeared in *Time* magazine and was gathered and presented through the hard work of reporters, writers, and editors, including Sally S. Stich, Julie Rawe, Leslie Whitaker, Dan Goodgame, Melissa August, Barbara Burgower-Hordern, Daren Fonda, Jyoti Thottam, Laura Koss-Feder, Betsy Rubiner, and Mary Sutter.

Introduction

Some sixty years ago a revolution began and it was anything but quiet, heralded by the wails and cries of the eighty-four million North Americans who would be born between 1946 and 1964. Making up a third of the continent's population, these baby boomers, as we came to be known, have been likened to a pig moving through a python—highly visible from start to finish. Our generation has dominated world culture since the end of World War II. Every time we have taken a step, the spotlight of the media has swiveled to illuminate us. By weight of sheer numbers we have amplified and intensified the importance of all our experiences, from the time we learned to use a baby bottle and then to read, play records, buy cars, vote, rent condos, and invest in the stock market. Whenever we reach any stage of life the issues that concern us—whether financial, interpersonal, or hormonal—become the dominant social, political, and economic themes of the time. The needs and desires of our massive generation become the primary concern of business as well as an unstoppable force shaping popular culture. We don't just experience life stages or consumer trends; we transform them.

1

- We didn't just eat food. Our migration through the teenage years spawned the fast-food industry, just as in recent years our health consciousness has sparked the creation of the health food and sports nutrition markets.

- We didn't just wear clothes. We transformed the fashion industry, leading such trends as denim and bell-bottoms in the teenage years; polyester in the '70s; and, most recently, the casual workplace.

- We didn't just date and marry. We transformed sex roles and practices, broke taboos of divorce, and transformed the traditional models of the nuclear family.

- We didn't just go to work. We transformed the workplace, breaking the corporate hierarchies and models of lifetime employment. The women of our generation were the first to seek equality in a formerly male-dominated workforce.

In our youth, we warned never to trust anyone over thirty. It was an expression of defiance for the rigid lifestyles and conventions of our parents' generation. Beginning in 2006, throughout North America every eight seconds another boomer will turn sixty; that's eleven thousand each day and four and a half million each year. Not a single boomer is left under age forty.

We are once again poised to defy convention. As we look downstream at retirement and old age, we don't like what we see. We're noticing that for the majority of today's older adults, the retirement dream is proving to be an unhappy and diminished period of life that is too often characterized by social isolation, loneliness, inertia, a sense of personal diminishment, and financial dependency.

The millions of us who make up the "youth generation," as we were called, are beginning to rewrite the rules; we are retiring retirement as our parents have known it in favor of something more youthful and exhilarating. In essence, we find ourselves at a social tipping point. Due to longer life spans, economic uncertainties, and the mass rejection of yesterday's model of old age, yesterday's model of retirement is being transformed. Instead of viewing the years ahead as a time of decline, retreat, and withdrawal, we are coming to see this as a terrific new opportunity to reevaluate our lives, consider new options, and chart new courses. The next chapter of our life's journey can be one of personal reinvention, financial liberation, career innovation, new relationships, and social and spiritual fulfillment.

As a psychologist, gerontologist, demographer, and author of ten previous books, Ken Dychtwald has spent more than thirty years exploring and envisioning the evolution of the baby boom into the Age Wave. As an award-winning journalist with twenty-five years in the field, Dan Kadlec has been insightfully covering the financial, social, and lifestyle implications of these issues first for *USA Today*, and for the past decade as a columnist and senior writer for *Time* magazine. In this book, we combine our more than fifty-five years of study, research, and reporting and share our best ideas about how to make the years ahead the best years of your life.

This book is the outgrowth of a meeting that was bound to occur: Ken, who has long been a valuable source for journalists, had just conducted a landmark study of the future of retirement and came across Dan's radar as Dan was preparing a *Time* cover story on trends that were conspiring to force boomers worldwide to work until they are eighty. We found ourselves agreeing on the unprecedented changes coming our way, and we agreed that few people were preparing sufficiently. We realized that those of us in our forties, fifties, and sixties today truly will be retirement's guinea pigs. We'll live long and in good health, and what sets us apart from our parents is that we know it—right now at an age when we are young enough to plan and get it right. However, too few of us seem to be taking this opportunity seriously. With that in mind, we set out to write a definitive guide to what comes next and how to make the most of it.

We are both optimists, so we wanted our message to be useful and uplifting as well as more visionary and comprehensive than anything you've ever read. Admittedly, scores of books and articles have addressed pieces of the broad topics we tackle here. But none takes adequate account of the new, youthful, engaged model of aging that we believe is unfolding. To that end, volumes have been written on where to retire for good weather and a low crime rate; but precious little has been written, as we have done in *The Power Years*, on exploring cities and towns that cater to retirees who still want to work, start a business, or feel fit enough to climb mountains. Tons of ink have been spilled describing how to save for retirement; little has been written, as we do here, about how to refit your financial requirements by downsizing, moving, and even keeping a job you love. We'll show you some new ways to have fun beyond bridge and golf, how to stay connected with your kids and grandkids beyond baking cookies or watching TV, how to fall in love again for real with your spouse or someone new, and how to leave a lasting legacy even if you've spent every dime you ever made.

These second chances are the essence of your power years. Don't be complacent. Plenty of curves lie ahead. So grab hold of the steering wheel, fasten your seat belt, and enjoy the ride.

1

Welcome to the Power Years

Do you long for a life without work or pressure in which your days are spent baking for the grandchildren or playing eighteen holes of golf in the morning, followed by a leisurely lunch and afternoon of bridge, then cocktails, a delicious early dinner, and a good movie? After all, that's how it worked for our grandparents and parents, isn't it? We grew up surrounded by this model of a leisure-filled later life.

Please forget everything you've been told. It's not your obligation to go away just because you're getting older. Nor is it your birthright to cede all responsibility to your community and mankind so that you may lead a life of leisure in retirement. Of course, you may choose these paths if you wish, but in our view that would be a mistake. Certainly there is no guarantee that you'll be able to afford a carefree romp through later life or even that you'll enjoy it if that's where you can afford to wind up. Reinventing yourself and *repowerment*—ramping up life where and when you choose and in ways that excite you, not winding down into obscurity—is the mold-shattering, exciting new stage that will come next for our generation.

While we've had our heads down toiling away these past few decades, spending more time than we might have envisioned at work and raising our children, the world has changed enormously. As we all know, the Internet, global trade, medical breakthroughs, and more are speeding up the pace of life even as life itself is being extended, posing new challenges in our careers and families. In this book, we cannot hope to deal with all the changes confronting our lives. Yet it's vitally important for each of us to appreciate just how different things really are and will become as we move into the next stage of life, a stage that we— the eighty-four million North Americans born between 1946 and 1964 as well as hundreds of millions more maturing adults around the world—will redefine as *the power years*.

Reinventing Retirement

The majority of our parents worked for one company all their lives. When their careers ended at age sixty-five, the norm was that they got a nice party and a gold watch and happily hopped on board a slow cruise into the sunset. Forty years of toil behind and the kids now grown, both Dad and Mom were done. They floated over the horizon, eagerly retreating to a life of leisure.

For their employers, it was a great deal. They got to bring in younger, more energetic, and less expensive labor.

For a lot of reasons, many of us won't have the same options that our parents had. For one thing, government and employee-sponsored entitlements have questionable futures, and the idea of early retirement, or even for many of us the idea of retirement at sixty-five, took a quantum leap backward when the global stock market bubble burst in 2000, eroding much of our savings and more than a few of our dreams.

Demographic trends threaten to foist an unprecedented labor shortage on the world economy. Companies of all sizes and shapes are going to want us to stick around longer and will be willing to provide us with a great deal more flexibility to do so. Meanwhile, our careers have been far more mobile. We've bounced among three, four, five, or more employers, often in as many cities, and we won't have been with any one of them long enough for a gold watch, much less the pension and wall-to-wall retirement health coverage that our parents might have been blessed with.

The slow, lazy cruise that our fathers and mothers eagerly signed up for turned out to be a little too slow and lazy. Look hard enough and you'll see that many of our parents have begun to rebel against the idea that they should fade away; they're going back to school and back to work, taking up writing or painting and otherwise reengaging with a society they had dropped out of. Throughout this book we will lean on the experiences of what we call Ageless Explorers, the growing number of leading-edge adults of our parents' generation and some from even farther back, to illustrate the changing nature of the power years. Our hope is that you'll find these anecdotes inspirational and that the glimmers they provide will meld into a beam of light that helps you navigate to—and through—your power years.

These years present a unique opportunity for us. The notion of staying in the game longer, of not having to step aside at a set age, will liberate us, setting us free to lead the lives we want to lead by staying engaged, vital, and youthful as long as we like. Opening before us is a whole new stage of life squeezed between our primary career years and a steadily retreating old age. Just as we moved from adolescence into adulthood three or four decades ago, we are now pushing into a whole new period of discovery and personal growth—what we call *middlescence*—as more and more of us make the most of the many fruitful decades that lie ahead.

Our generation is coming to realize that we will have numerous decades to live past the age commonly thought to be the time to stop working. What we do with that time will set us apart from all previous generations.

This book is for people like you who are beginning to contemplate what comes next and how to make the most of it. Make no mistake—this is not a retirement guide. It's about *unretiring*— about how to shed your dated preconceptions about life after forty, fifty, or sixty and stay in the game in ways you'll find satisfying and invigorating. Money is important, and we'll deal with that critical issue in chapter 7. But that's where this book stops being like anything you've read before. Countless opportunities are developing to let you live all aspects of your life to the fullest—from staying connected with your kids and grandkids (and, eventually, your great-grandkids) to choosing emerging housing designs and lifestyles for a new, active time in your life with fewer responsibilities; from finding love all over again with your spouse (or someone new, should you be searching) to going back to school for the fun of it; from where, how, and why to make new friends to where and why you should pick up stakes and move to a city or town that will let you live and thrive as you always dreamed.

We'll discover new passions and explore long-dormant desires. We'll stay active by working longer or volunteering, by trying our hand at writing or painting or running a small business, and our continued involvement will promote our well-being and prove a vital resource to the communities in which we live.

You are on a far different life track from that of your parents; you just may not fully understand it yet. But you soon will, and this book is meant to help you as you ramp up your learning curve.

On a recent vacation with his family in Orlando, Florida, Dan was staying at a wonderful resort, the Gaylord, where he observed an apparent oddity that both encouraged and, at least initially, dumbfounded him. The hotel had two equally spacious and convenient swimming pools on either side of the grounds. One was designated as a quiet zone for rest-seeking grown-ups and marked "No One under 18 Allowed." That pool area might as well have been a mausoleum—not a single person was in the water. The other pool, by contrast, was overrun with raucous teens and quite a few bawling toddlers. What stunned Dan was that many of the mature adults he would have expected to find at the quiet pool had opted away from that morguelike environ, preferring—even in some cases with no children or grandchildren in sight—the lively atmosphere at the pool bustling with the energy of youth.

Which pool will you choose in the years ahead?

When is the last time you seriously asked yourself what you will do with the rest of your life? Is there a second or a third career you'd like to explore? A small business you want to start? Do you want to study art or open a bed and breakfast? Have you dreamed of taking up acting or going to cooking school? Where should you live for the perfect combination of weather, fun, friendships, family, lovers, intellectual stimulation, and lifestyle? What will all that free time do to our marriages and other relationships? Where and how will we live? What will keep our minds active and our lives relevant? Will this be the worst period of our lives—or could it possibly be the best? Most important: what choices must we make now to ensure the kind of extended life after career that we have always envisioned?

You can't get there if you don't think about it, yet few people ask the key questions. We assume that we can deal with these issues when the time comes, reasoning that as long as we manage to save a lot of money, everything will work out. But this is backward thinking. A big pile of money shouldn't be your primary goal. Who you want to be, what you want to feel, and what you want to do with your power years are the critical considerations, and from those spring the types of choices and trade-offs you'll need to consider.

You wouldn't think of building a house without a plan. You wouldn't go on vacation without thinking through your itinerary and even your wardrobe. So why leave your power years to chance? Even if you're not wealthy, you can enjoy an active, fulfilling, and youthful next stage of life by understanding your goals and creating a carefully thought-out plan that makes those goals possible. In this book, we will guide you through every aspect of this blueprint and show you a wide range of choices and possibilities you may never have considered.

As we step over the threshold into maturity, we will transform the stage of later life known as retirement into something that squares with our generation's desire to work, play, and love on our own terms, staying young in mind and body, and engaging in new pursuits without becoming bogged down with too many numbing obligations. With greater energy and drive, higher expectations for our later years, and a greater willingness to repeatedly reinvent ourselves than any previous generation, perhaps we'll reshape work into something that we can do three days a week, or eight months each year, or seven years per decade. And with extended longevity, why wait until maturity for a long break? Why not take time off along the way? Instead of being stuck on a one-career path for life, why not go back to school, learn some new skills, and reinvent ourselves again and again?

The Baby Boom Becomes the Age Wave

What we're naming the power years has also been called by some our *third age*, a concept derived from the European tradition of adult education. This view holds that there are three ages of man, each with its own special focus, challenges, and opportunities. In the first age, from birth to about thirty, our primary tasks of life are biological development, learning, and survival. During most of human history, the average life expectancy wasn't much longer than the end of the first age, and as a result, the entire thrust of society was oriented toward these basic drives.

In the second age, from about thirty to sixty, our concerns focus on forming a family, parenting, and work. We apply the lessons we learned during the first age to these responsibilities. Until very recently, most people didn't live much beyond the second age. But with today's longer life expectancies, new generations of youthful, open-minded, and high-spirited men and women are not interested in fading into the sunset at sixty.

A third age, which spans the period from sixty to ninety (and longer), is unfolding ahead of us. This is a less-pressured period in which we can further develop our intellect, imagination, emotional maturity, and wisdom. This is also a period when we can give something back to society based on the lessons, resources, and experiences we have accumulated over a lifetime. We need not be social outcasts, but instead can assume the role of a living bridge between yesterday and tomorrow, and in this way play a critical role that no other group is as well suited to perform.

In recent decades, a small but growing number of older adults have been rejecting the social pressure to "act their age." They have been rebelling against ageist stereotypes and seeking to remain productive, involved, and late blooming well into their mature years. They are everywhere—within our families, among our friends, and in our communities: the executive who becomes a high school teacher; the grandmother who goes back to college or who writes her first book; the accountant who becomes an artist. Ask them when they think they'll start to feel elderly inside, and they'll probably say *never*!

In his book *The Virtues of Aging*, Jimmy Carter lit the repowerment path in a single phrase at the end of this telling passage: "In one of her hour-long special interviews, Barbara Walters covered all the aspects of my life, from the farm to submarines, from business to the governor's mansion, service in the White

House, and from president back home to Plains. Then she asked me a question that required some serious thought: 'Mr. President, you have had a number of exciting and challenging careers. What have been your best years?' After a few moments I responded with absolute certainty: '*Now* is the best time of all.'"

If the past fifty years of boomer evolution have taught us anything, it is this: as we enter each new life stage we keep what we like and replace the rest, like remodeling a house.

We'll be moving and experimenting with new lifestyles. As we stay in the game longer both socially and economically, we'll reshape family and community life. One breathtaking finding from the Merrill Lynch New Retirement Survey surfaced when we asked boomers how they would describe themselves. Ten times as many survey respondents said they "put others first" as said "put themselves first." A far cry from our rambunctious teenage years and our swinging single period, we're now focused on keeping our marriages strong, on trying our best to raise healthy and happy children, and on caregiving our parents (the average boomer now has more parents than children to care for). The *me* generation has grown up to be a *we* generation. This attitude shift will reshape philanthropy and volunteerism and may very well be the cornerstone of the new retirement values. Today's retirees have the lowest volunteer rate in the country, while those our age who are actively helping out in our kids' schools and in community churches/synagogues through various philanthropic activities actually have the highest volunteer rate. If this desire to make a difference continues into retirement, we may see a huge change in the role of retirees overall—from taking to giving.

With the right insight and planning, we'll be able to merge what we most enjoy in our youth—energy, freedom, flexibility, health, and personal growth—with the good things that come with age, things such as experience, perspective, wisdom, and depth. One thing is clear: as our massive numbers ultimately catch the wave, the ripples will stretch far and wide.

The Seven Reasons These Are the Power Years

Why are these becoming the power years? Here are seven reasons why the rest of your life has more potential than you may have considered:

1. We'll Be Living Longer and Healthier

In 1800, the average life expectancy was less than forty years. By 1900, when one in five babies didn't make it to their fifth birthday and common causes of death were diarrhea, influenza, pneumonia, and tuberculosis, life expectancy at birth was just forty-seven years. Thanks to advances in public health, nutrition, and wellness-oriented lifestyles, today the average lifetime has stretched to more than seventy-seven years in all of the modernized nations of the world. Japan has one of the highest expectancies: seventy-eight years for men and eighty-four for women, for an overall average of eighty-one years. The tiny nation of Andorra, squeezed between France and Spain, tops the world charts in this regard with newborn boys likely to reach eighty-one and newborn girls expected to make it to eighty-seven, for an overall average of eighty-four years. The United States is far down the list, with an overall life expectancy of seventy-seven—behind Singapore (eighty-two), Switzerland, Sweden, Canada, and Italy (all of which have expected average life spans at birth of eighty years). If you've already made it to fifty, you can expect to live at least until your mid-eighties, and thanks to impending scientific breakthroughs, these numbers will keep increasing.

We will live longer and grow old later in life than any previous generation. Incredibly, two-thirds of all those who have made it to age sixty-five in the history of mankind are today walking the earth. We're not just living longer, we are also in better health and enjoy greater youthfulness and vitality. There are more fifty- and sixty-year-olds running marathons, buying Harleys, starting new careers, going to rock concerts, and getting facelifts than ever before. Our increasing longevity and good health, coupled with our natural desire to remain youthful, are the greatest forces behind the power years. But technology and modern medicine are playing vital roles as well. Impending miracle treatments could help us beat everything from arthritis to Alzheimer's, and the arrival of the information age is taking much of the physical toil out of work and other pursuits.

The upshot is that great numbers of people—not just exceptions—are able to work and play as they like far longer than anyone might have expected.

2. The Cyclic Lifeplan Will Replace the Outmoded Linear Model

Greater longevity and vitality will change core patterns of society. When people lived just thirty or forty years, life followed a well-defined linear path. We grew up, went to school, worked hard while marrying and rearing a family, and then we died. Everything had its place, and life was too short for second chances. Increased longevity transforms this model. All around us, the linear path is being replaced by something more flexible. As Maddy Dychtwald explained in her book *Cycles*, now we can cycle in and out of careers—interspersing periods of rest and retraining. We may end up working longer, but rather than saving all of our leisure for the end of our lives, regular breaks throughout adulthood will become commonplace. Formal sabbaticals and informal work leaves will be part of every major company's standard package of benefits.

The landmark New Retirement Survey that Ken directed in 2004 with Merrill Lynch was based on interviews with more than three thousand boomers (www.totalmerrill.com/retirement). The study found that only 17 percent of them said they intended to stop working for pay forever in their next stage of life. A whopping 42 percent reported that they hoped to cycle in and out of work and leisure for extended periods throughout life; 16 percent expected to continue working part-time; 13 percent were planning on starting their own business; and 6 percent fully intended to keep working full-time right through their retirement years. Incredibly, of the 76 percent who intended to continue working in some fashion, more than half were hoping to do so in a completely new career or line of work!

Further, when asked why so many wanted to stay involved with work, the overwhelming response was not money. Instead, two of three said the main reason was to stay mentally active. Members of our highly educated and productive generation simply don't want to live a life of intellectual stagnation and mental irrelevance.

3. We'll Have a Big—and Growing— Pool of Role Models

How about John Glenn going back into space, and what about Sumner Redstone, who in his eighties is chairman of Viacom, and Rupert Murdoch, who at seventy-four is chairman of News Corporation? They are running two of the world's largest media empires as though they expect to be around to see their visions realized decades hence. Who knows? Maybe they will be.

Warren Buffett remains the world's greatest investor midway through his seventies. *People* magazine named Sean Connery the sexiest man alive in 1989 when he was fifty-nine. Sophia Loren is pretty terrific in her seventh decade of life, too. Joe Paterno, at seventy-seven, signed a four-year contract extension to coach the vaunted Penn State football team.

Late achievement, while multiplying in frequency, isn't altogether new. Grandma Moses didn't start painting until she was almost eighty. Groucho Marx launched a new career as a television-show host at sixty-five. George Bernard Shaw was at work on a new play when he died at ninety-four. Galileo published his masterpiece *Dialogue Concerning the Two New Sciences* at seventy-four. Noah Webster was seventy when he published *An American Dictionary of the English Language*. Frank Lloyd Wright designed the Guggenheim Museum in New York at ninety-one. Mahatma Gandhi was seventy-two when he completed successful negotiations with Britain for India's independence. I. M. Pei was seventy-eight when he designed the Rock and Roll Hall of Fame and Museum in Cleveland. Picasso painted *The Rape of the Sabines* at eighty-one. Golda Meir was prime minister of Israel from ages seventy to seventy-six. Jessica Tandy was eighty when she won her first Oscar for *Driving Miss Daisy*. Mary Baker Eddy was eighty-seven when she founded the *Christian Science Monitor*. At ninety-three, Lillian Gish starred in *The Whales of August* seventy-two years after starring in the silent film *Birth of a Nation*. At ninety-four, conductor Leopold Stokowski signed a six-year recording contract. At a hundred, Ichijirou Araya climbed Mount Fuji.

In their day, these remarkable men and women may have been considered highly unusual. But these Ageless Explorers have carved new trails ahead of us and represent the first wave of maturity pioneers. We baby boomers will be next, and we'll turn this thorny trail into a superhighway. Many of us are already thinking ahead. Joel Levinson, fifty-one, has begun to picture his power years as a real-estate investor. He's enjoyed a fruitful career in the advertising business and has run his own agency for the past decade. But he doesn't want to do that forever, and sees real estate as an exciting challenge and a way to build both an income stream for life and his net worth. Joel is in a great spot. He's reaching financial freedom ahead of his own expectations, and he has already begun mapping out how he'll break into the real-estate game, which he has been quietly passionate about for years.

"Every time we plan a vacation, I build in time to go alone and scout out properties in the area," he says. "I lov comparing values and studying what makes one place worth more than another. And lately I've begun to bore friends who are even remotely connected to the real-estate industry— lawyers, brokers, investors—with all my talk about getting into the game."

Joel says he's just days away from making his first invest- ment. "Have been for years," he jokes. "There's always another book to read or another property to look at, so I've been slow to pull the trigger. And I'm wary that prices may be a bit inflated these days." But he figures all of his hours studying markets will pay off when he finally buys that first property. Besides, he's enjoyed every minute of his research.

Joel still has two kids at home, so he's in no rush to give up his primary, high-earning career. "The longer I wait, and the more I study, the greater chances of success I'll have when I finally start buying," he says. "I don't intend to take big risks. I'll buy one at a time and keep reinvesting the profits, and see how it works out. I figure I can minimize any chances that I'll lose money. I'll probably do very well, and if nothing else I'll enjoy how I'm spending my time."

4. We'll Be Wiser about What Matters

Having climbed much of the mountain, you now have a pretty good view of life. As we accumulate and make sense of life's les- sons, most of us have come to appreciate that the joy that money alone brings is fleeting, and that true happiness revolves around love, relationships, and our sense of fulfillment at work and at play. Most of us reach this basic understanding in our middle years—sometimes precipitated by the death of a parent, our kids leaving home, or the failure of a career or marriage. But for the most part, by the time we're fifty and still young enough to shape

...lerstand that money, while it's important,
...happiness.

...eaded a massive international study with
...he Future of Retirement (www.HSBC.com/
...ement). When eleven thousand people of all ages
...ons including Brazil, Canada, China, France, Hong
...India, Japan, Mexico, the United Kingdom, and the
...ted States were asked what they believed contributed most
...o achieving a happy old age, the overwhelming first choice was
"loving family and friends." Thanks to the additional longevity
we'll be experiencing, we will have both the time and the wisdom to realize what brings true happiness.

In a series of surveys over the past twenty years, *Forbes* magazine has asked people to rate their happiness on a scale of 1 to 7, with 1 being "not at all satisfied with my life" and 7 being "completely satisfied." No surprise, those on the *Forbes* 400 list of wealthiest people in the world clocked in with a healthy average response of 5.8. But so did the modest-living Inuit people of frigid northern Greenland, and so did the cattle-herding Masai of Kenya, who live in huts with no electricity or running water.

Tom Hagan of Covington, Ohio, sold his pharmacy business at age fifty-six. But he didn't retire. He remains employed in the industry; he simply gave up the headaches and rewards of ownership. "The secret to life is being fulfilled," Hagan says. "It has nothing to do with money. I have friends who are worth $50 million who are miserable. They hate their wives; they hate their children. I love my life. I'm still working, and I plan to work until I die. I love my new job. It keeps my mind active. I couldn't imagine sitting around and watching TV every day."

5. We'll Have New Freedoms

The kids are gone or soon will be. College and the house are paid for—well, mostly paid for. In any case, you probably have amassed a fair amount of home equity, and hopefully you've been stashing some money in a retirement plan at work. It's not just that your kids' schooling and the mortgage are mostly taken care of. Things like braces and summer camp and all the things you put in your house are largely paid for; you don't need a lot more stuff. With many of your biggest parenting-related financial obligations coming to an end, you'll be endowed with greater freedom to do the things you've always wanted. Meanwhile, your busy schedule is beginning to let up, providing you with a windfall of free time that will let you take on new challenges or pursue hidden passions and long-suppressed dreams.

And because the economy will want to simultaneously prevent a brain drain and declining consumption by keeping all of us earning and spending longer, it will become easier to stay at work or start a new career. The vacuum of workers maturing means that older adults will be in demand and more able to choose our own schedules, and still remain valuable. With the rise of flextime and part-time schedules and contract and project jobs and job sharing, there are millions of exciting paths for us to explore in the work world—throughout the world. With online universities, we can retrain at home or pursue a life as a writer or artist or some other dream.

6. We'll Still Have Clout in the Marketplace

Our huge numbers and often free-spending ways have ensured throughout our lifetime that anyone with something to sell would be inclined to tailor it to our wants and needs. Our demographic and financial wells of influence won't run dry as we mature. We'll live longer and healthier and remain active consumers. Meanwhile, as a generation, our wealth will continue to multiply. Already, today's fifty-plus men and women are the principal buyers of luxury cars, leisure travel, and high-end gifts and jewelry. We own 40 percent of all mutual funds and 60 percent of all annuities. While we are just 30 percent of the population, we control more than 70 percent of all of the wealth and account for more than 50 percent of consumer spending. As we mature and collectively inherit an estimated $20 trillion, we will be as cherished as ever in the marketplace.

Advertisers will need to break free of their addiction to youth. Many wrongly believe that all adults have already chosen the brands they will stick with for life, while young people have yet to choose their cola, sneaker, cell phone, or whatever. This flawed view will stop paying off; marketers will increasingly come to realize that at fifty or sixty we not only have money to spend but also are eager to ditch our old lipstick for the latest colors. As we age, we will remain interested in new adventures and experiences, and we will spend freely to reach our full potential in the power years.

In the years ahead, watch for growth in industries such as the following:

- specialty diagnosis and treatment centers for particular body parts, such as the eyes, ears, muscles, bones, or nervous system

- therapeutically cloned kidneys, livers, lungs, hearts, skin, blood, and bones for tune-up or replacement

- nutraceuticals engineered with macro- and micronutrients to fight aging

- cosmeceutical rejuvenation therapies for both men and women

- antiaging spas

- high-tech exercise gear and equipment programmed to precisely train users to build stronger, healthier, and more youthful bodies

- smart acoustic systems in telephones, radios, and TVs that customize signals to accommodate the auditory range of each user's ears

- Silver Seals—for-hire teams of elders with various problem-solving talents who are deployed to fix difficult community or business issues

- lifelong learning programs at colleges, universities, churches, and community centers and on cable TV and the Internet

- "retirement zone" stores featuring products and technologies appealing to older adults with free time

- adventure travel services that send older adults to off-the-beaten-trail locations

- mature employment and career transition coordinators; experience agents—similar to travel agents—who can be commissioned to orchestrate any type of request, whether it's a party, learning program, psychotherapy, sabbatical, travel adventure, spiritual retreat, introduction to new friends, dates, or business partnerships

- mature dating services to help the tens of millions of single mature women and men find new relationships

- longevity-oriented communities for health-minded elders

- intergenerational communes

- Club Med–like residences for those who enjoy active social programming

- urban arts retirement communities that focus on cultural pursuits

- university-based intergenerational housing for people who desire lifelong learning

- hedonism complexes for mature swingers

- multinational time-share clubs for those who aren't interested in settling down in one location

- long-term-care insurance financing to provide security against the possibility of late-life chronic health problems

- longevity insurance that, rather than paying an individual's family in case of early death, provides financial support for people who live very long

- estate management and trust services to help families manage the $20+ trillion inheritance cascade that is about to occur

- reverse mortgages to help people who are cash-poor but "brick-rich."

7. We'll Be Open to Change

Personal growth and self-improvement are the new order, and as this mind-set blossoms, it will open the doors to fulfillment and achievement that might otherwise have been stifled.

The world of continuing education may best illustrate the appetites of a generation that loves to learn and grow. Already, a thriving adult-education industry has begun to flourish, including magazines, books, audio, video, Internet learning programs, and adult-education seminars, workshops, and courses. About forty million adults participate in one or more educational activities each year. As the need to continuously upgrade skills becomes a requirement, lifelong learning will become commonplace. In response, colleges and universities have begun to aggressively pursue adult students. *USA Today* recounted: "admission officers and financial-aid directors from campuses across the USA echo the message: Older students are as desirable—often more so—as the traditional 18-to-24 college crowd. And they're just as eligible for grants and loans as their younger brethren. Adults, they say, are better motivated, usually have educational goals in focus, and have experiences to share with younger students."

A quiet revolution is occurring. Students over age thirty-five were just 5.5 percent of higher-education enrollment in 1970; today 22 percent of all college students are over thirty-five. Meanwhile, the percentage of adults age sixty-six to seventy-four who enrolled in at least one adult-education course more than doubled between 1990 and 2000, to 20 percent. Retirees represent 25 percent of the ten thousand University of Chicago students taking noncredit courses in the arts and sciences. The trend toward older students will build as adults of all ages seek to upgrade their knowledge through formal university programs, correspondence courses, and employer-provided retraining. This is a worldwide phenomenon. In one respect, Canadians are leading the way, with 6 percent of all adults enrolled in one or more university courses. South Korea ranks second, followed by Australia and then the United States. But New Zealand, Finland, Norway, Spain, Ireland, and France aren't far behind.

Aging Rocks

Being a grandpa or a grandma will rock if we plan for those later years now, doing what we must to be able to stay active, in tune, and in touch. Is it possible to stay hip when we've reached the age of grandparenting? Ask Mick Jagger, Ringo Starr, Paul McCartney, or Keith Richards. All of them have kids with kids. They still rock, and none has lost an ounce of cool. When asked about his age, Richards recently commented, "Getting old is a fascinating thing. The older you get, the older you want to get."

We have grown up equating retirement with old age. But with the oldest of our generation starting to celebrate sixty, that's beginning to change. We aren't looking to be old or to wind down. We're looking to begin a whole new life when we reach our fifties and sixties. Having a positive outlook and understanding that life's next chapter is just that—not the beginning of the end of life—are vital to making it fun and fulfilling.

The power years are coming, and we want to be your guides.

2

New Ways to Have Fun

One of the great things about what comes next is that most of us can expect to end up with plenty of time for fun and with the resources to enjoy that time. We understand that emerging financial trends will make it difficult to amass a sizable stake, and we recognize that many of us will continue to work part-time or flextime for a variety of reasons. But if you take the time now to think through all of the options presented in this book, your power years can be grander and far more enjoyable than you may imagine.

For our grandparents who worked hard and may have died young, leisure amounted to Sunday afternoons with the family and a yearly one-week trip down- or upstate. Our parents broadened the model, daring to eat out once in a while but generally restricting leisure to short weekend bursts and perhaps a two-week family trip each year.

Our generation will morph leisure as completely as the idea of retirement itself. We'll embark on wilderness adventures and exotic travel—not from the safe sanctum of a cruise-ship deck or tour bus, but in the classrooms, urban centers, jungles, and fields of remote lands as part of experiential vacations, volunteer work, and cultural study. We'll scour the Internet and pore through catalogs for the kind of fun and creative free time that holds special appeal just to us. We'll use recreation to strengthen our most important relationships and make some new friends along the way. Liberated from parenting and full-time work, we'll roam the world and search deep inside ourselves for new experiences, new thrills, new awarenesses, and new beginnings.

Already, dozens of companies have emerged to serve our longing to reignite our sense of discovery and adventure by trudging through a rain forest, observing wild Africa, debating global politics in a lively classroom, or simply relaxing on the beach with plenty of amenities. Thousands more will appear as we collectively create a huge commercial market for innovative leisure concepts that are at once youthful in nature and geared to more seasoned appetites.

In the New Retirement Survey, when boomers were asked what they were looking forward to most in the next phase of their lives, the response "having more fun" outranked every other choice on the list. That was followed by reducing stress, more time with our spouse, traveling, more time with our children and grandchildren, simplifying our lives, hobbies, rest and relaxation, time to focus on myself, and enhancing my spiritual side.

Are you ready to have fun again, explore your deepest passions, pursue your wildest dreams, tap your hidden potentials? It's probably hard to imagine. In recent decades we have come to almost universally describe daily life with words such as "frenzied," "overextended," and "exhausted." Most of us are part of dual-income couples or hardworking single parents struggling to balance work and family, and finding only an occasional weekend for a little R&R. Racing around to meet everyone's needs, behind in the bills, the light at the end of the tunnel may seem no bigger than a lit match in an ocean of dark. Recently Ken needed to talk with his lawyer about a business contract. He dialed the number and when he answered the phone, Ken sensed that he was in the middle of a hassle. Ken asked "Is this a good time to talk?" to which his lawyer answered "Hey, the last good time to talk was in college." He's not alone.

If it feels like work has taken over our lives, well, it has. Officially, the average workweek has long hovered at about thirty-four hours. But that's a misleading figure. If you work in the massive financial services industry, your workweek averages fifty-five hours. For top executives, regardless of industry, the workweek runs sixty to seventy hours, reports Catalyst, a research and consulting group. For dual-career couples with children under age eighteen, combined weekly work hours grew from eighty-one in 1977 to ninety-one in 2002, according to the Families and Work Institute. We are rich in things, but time has come to be our scarcest resource. Says Harvard economist Juliet B. Schor, author of *The Overworked American*: "The shrinkage of leisure, experienced by nearly all types of Americans, has created a profound structural crisis in time."

It's brought us to this: on a routine workday in January 2004, some ten inches of snow fell on New York City, and in a turn that veteran city dwellers deemed wimpy, tens of thousands of hard-core workers took a snow day. Subways were running but empty; offices were open but ran on skeleton crews. Ten inches of snow isn't exactly crippling in the wintry Northeast. A dozen years ago hearty New Yorkers would have fought through it without hesitation. What made this day different? In our 24-7 lives we're being worked to death. "We're just tired and think we need an extra day off," Carol Peligian, a Manhattan artist, explained to the *New York Times*.

In a comprehensive survey of seventy-five hundred workers called The New Employer/Employee Equation conducted by Ken and Age Wave in collaboration with the Concours Group, when asked which mattered more—paid maternity leave, flexible work schedules, or additional paid vacation, workers over-whelmingly ranked additional paid vacation as their biggest desire. This response received more than twice the votes as either a more flexible work schedule or paid maternity leave.

Even weekends off don't offer the relief they should. After a hectic workweek, our free time is often consumed by house chores, parenting responsibilities, and, increasingly, more work. That report the boss needs by Monday was put off last week because of all the things that needed doing then and, well, we could always get to it on Saturday. There's been a lot of hype about how technology can give you a better quality of life. But part of what that means is that through the Web and our cell phones, we're never out of touch. How often have you been in the midst of some leisure pursuit only to have it ruined by a work-related phone call or e-mail? And how frequently have you seen a friend supposedly enjoying quality time with family while multitasking with phone calls or instant messaging?

As founder and CEO of outplacement consultancy Challenger, Gray & Christmas, John Challenger stays on top of workplace trends. He sees a real danger in our culture of endless work. "People burn out," he says, and inevitably, burnout leads to turnover. "No company can afford to lose its best people by running them so hard they ultimately move on. That means giving them room to breathe." The workaholic culture in America is legendary. Americans don't get anywhere near as much time off as most Europeans. France and Germany pretty much shut down during August. In France, there's a mandated thirty-five-hour workweek, and workers spend 30 percent less time at the office than Americans. A survey from the American Management Association shows that 58 percent of managers plan to stay in touch with their workplaces while on vacation, and only 31% take more than a week off at a time. On average, Americans take off only ten days a year with pay versus thirty in Germany and Spain, twenty-five in the United Kingdom and

Australia, eighteen in Japan, and fifteen in China. The World Tourism Organization says Italians average an astounding forty-two vacation days a year. Yet these countries maintain high rates of productivity. Could it be that their employees work more effectively and are less stressed due to a saner balance between work and play?

It hasn't always been like this. The ancient Greeks considered new experiences in their nonworking hours to be the main purpose of life. Work was a necessity normally performed by slaves and serfs while leisure was an activity engaged in by the privileged and enlightened classes. In Greek culture it was work that was defined by what it wasn't: leisure. This is clear in their vocabulary. The Greek word for leisure is *schole*. The word for work is *ascholia*, which means the absence of leisure. The Greeks prioritized leisure. We've turned the tables, and while the reversal has brought us many fancy things, it may also be robbing us of time to discover ourselves, nurture relationships, and just enjoy life.

In our power years, we will have more time to goof off, read some good books, learn to paint, enjoy a fine dinner with close friends, make love, go sailing, or just kick back and enjoy a beautiful sunrise than during any previous period of our lives. We will have the mental perspective, the financial wherewithal, and the emotional depth to finally create a better work-play balance. We may have a few more wrinkles, but with them comes the realization that material ambition does not equal personal fulfillment.

In the drought and heat of Berkeley, California, in the summer of 1991, fires ravaged the hillsides near where Ken lives. As flames swept through the area, residents hurriedly packed their cars with their most precious things and evacuated. What did they take? Not their large-screen TVs or their expensive dining room set, that's for sure. As they fled, they chose to save pictures and souvenirs of interesting moments in their life. These were their most cherished possessions. It's the experiences we share with those around us that ultimately mean the most to us and make us feel most alive. In our power years we will have time to focus on the joy in relationships and the fun and sense of discovery we get from pleasurable experiences. Our new leisure activities will be more intellectually stimulating, socially engaging, vigorous, and adventuresome. Just as we helped launch the backpacking and youth hosteling movements of the 1960s and '70s, and the fitness and spa trends of the 1980s and '90s, we'll bring to our power years a long-suppressed appetite for fun and adventure.

More Free Time Than Ever Before

Millions of us have already begun to taste what life is like with more discretionary time. Still working but with children in college or having moved out for good, we have begun to discover that a critical turning point to the power years isn't necessarily when we quit our primary career; it's that seminal moment when we become "empty nesters." Think about the rare occasions over the past twenty years or so when your kids were visiting Grandma for the weekend or off at camp and you could do anything you wanted. What did you do? Take a carefree trip? Enjoy a rare, spontaneous sexual encounter with your spouse? Or perhaps prepare a five-course dinner on a whim? That's what life will be like every day in your power years; you'll be able to do whatever you want, whenever you feel like it.

For many, empty nesting—not necessarily retiring from work—provides our first serious taste of freedom. This is when we change when and for how long we take our vacations, what we do with seven free evenings each week, how we remodel our homes or relocate. And given that we'll have increasing workplace flexibility, taking off weeks, months, or years at a time, managing discretionary time will become just as important as managing discretionary income.

Originally, the term "empty nest" had a negative connotation, which is how it was linked to the word "syndrome." Empty-nest syndrome was thought to be a form of depression suffered by mothers who after devoting years of their life to raising children felt desolate and abandoned. Some mothers and fathers still suffer bouts of empty-nest syndrome. For inspiration and camaraderie log on to www.emptynestmoms.com.

In recent years, however, the "syndrome" aspect of becoming an empty nester has receded to the background as Ageless Explorers have begun to embrace the years when they are free to play and do as they want again. This shift is evident in the redecoration of homes. "Empty-nester homes of the past were the same home as when they were a full nest, [but] the extra bedroom would become the sewing room," says Todd Lawson, architect and coauthor of *The House to Ourselves: Reinventing Home Once the Kids Are Grown*. Now, he says, "It's everything under the sun."

"Empty-nesters are really prime for remodeling," says Kathe Ostrom, president of the design-build firm C. N. Ostrom & Son. "They go, 'It's my turn.' In this new phase, maybe there's more time for hobbies. People are working from home because it's peaceful and there's a spare room where they can set up an office. And they have more money to spend, and they're looking to have more fun—doing the spa bathroom . . . putting in the steam showers and the exercise equipment, having a place that they can call theirs."

Empty nesters aren't just remodeling, they're also buying sexy sports cars, signing up for weekend yoga workshops at Esalen Institute in Big Sur, taking classes in film production at the Open Exchange free university in New York City, attending wine tasting programs at the Calistoga Ranch in Napa, volunteering to build homes for Habitat for Humanity all over the world, learning to cook exotic new foods, working out at the local gym, and attending shows and theatrical performances in droves.

Take More Time Off Along the Way

While we're on the subject of leisure, rather than save all of your leisure for the end of your life, why not take some time off from work along the way? The lockstep model of forty years of uninterrupted work followed by twenty to thirty years of recreation is dissolving. To strike a more satisfying work-life balance, consider taking an informal work leave, a paid sabbatical, and more frequent and more extended vacations. It's getting easier all the time. Companies such as Xerox and Arrow Electronics have institutionalized flexible work schedules and sabbaticals. More companies are hopping aboard every day to retain good workers and build morale.

After John Tronco married in 2001, he and his wife spent eighteen days in Italy and France, two days unpacking when he got back home to Charlotte, North Carolina, and then a week in Kiawah, South Carolina. When he returned to his job he still had three weeks of paid vacation remaining. How? He took advantage of a generous work-leave policy at Charlotte-based Spectrum Properties, a commercial real-estate company where he is a marketing representative. Paid sabbaticals are de rigueur at Spectrum. After five years, employees get four consecutive weeks of paid leave on top of their regular vacation. After the next five years, they get another month-long paid break, and so on for every five years they're with the company.

"On my first sabbatical, I stayed home and landscaped my yard," said Carol King, fifty-eight, an executive assistant at Spectrum. "That's not going to Africa and helping out the world, but it was very rejuvenating for me." That's exactly the point, says John Boylan, executive vice president and head of the Raleigh office. "We don't want someone to go take a second job for that month to make extra money. We want people to go away and come back excited."

Have Some Fun

You've worked hard. You've had your moments of leisure, but life really has not been a barrel of laughs in recent decades. Why not take the opportunity to indulge in something that brings you joy just for joy's sake?

Curt and Jeannie Schryer looked forward to the day that Curt could wind up his job with the U.S. Department of Energy. They saved diligently, putting most of their nest egg in the stock market but being careful to stash some in ultrasafe U.S. Savings Bonds. When the stock market went south in 2000 it hurt, but it didn't derail their plans because they had enough savings to fund their retirement without selling stocks before the market began to recover. They moved fifteen miles outside of Honolulu, where they enjoy breathtaking mountain and ocean views. Curt, fifty-eight, goes golfing three times a week; he and his wife travel often, and they recently hiked through Greece and cycled through Portugal. Both are enjoying the good life just as they had always envisioned, and they have no regrets.

There's nothing wrong with a healthy dose of relaxation, especially in the months or years immediately after scaling back or quitting your primary career. You have earned a break, so take one. There is no shortage of businesses to help you get away from it all, from basic travel services firms to online planners such as www.expedia.com and www.orbitz.com and www.travelocity .com. More exotic planners include Geographic Expeditions (www.geoex.com), which specializes in custom luxury travel to places such as Tibet, Nepal, Mongolia, Vietnam, Burma, and Patagonia; and Corniche Travel (www.corniche.com), which provides private villas in places such as Tuscany and Provence. Go ahead and enjoy yourself. There will be plenty of time to light new fires in your power years.

Athletic and rejuvenation programs, auto racing courses, cooking workshops, and rock and roll fantasy camps are popping up everywhere to offer us the chance to have a blast doing fun things. These camps are specifically designed for active adults, and as we enter our power years there will be an increasing emphasis on tailoring these camps to our needs. For a complete listing of what's out there, visit www.grownupcamps.com. With the slogan "Why should kids have all the fun?" it lists more than seven thousand weekend and week-long experiences, from business and film to dance, writing, and horseback riding.

For Sandy and Ken Piper of Geneva, Ohio, the fantasy Ballroom Vermont Dance Camp changed their life together. Sandy, forty-five, had been intrigued with ballroom dancing for years before meeting Ken, fifty-six. Her own parents had met on a dance floor, and she recalls falling in love with the spectacle of ballrooms as a child. The Pipers have gone to the one-week camp in Killington, Vermont, for seven consecutive years to mingle with dance champs such as Bob Powers and Julia Gorchakova, and, says Sandy, "I don't see any reason to stop." She and her husband view the camp as a way to relax and at the same time get some exercise. But more importantly, Sandy says, "Ballroom dancing gives us a passion that we share together and helps us grow closer. A lot of couples go their separate ways after the kids are gone. I didn't want that to happen to us. Dancing is such an enjoyable way to spend time together. It's really been perfect for us." They have made many new friends on the dance floor and at camp.

If you dream of laying down a few tracks with fellow rocker wannabes in the company of folks such as Roger Daltry, Leslie West, and Mark Farner, check out www.rockandrollfantasy camp.com. That's what Fred Dawson of Wilmington, Delaware, did, and he couldn't be happier. Dawson, fifty-five, loves his Hammond B-3 keyboard and went to a rock camp in Los Angeles several years ago to play alongside the likes of George Thoroughgood and Spencer Davis. "In my misspent youth I played in a garage band with moderate success," Dawson says, "I put it all down for decades to become a financial adviser, and I just wanted to go touch the cloth of people who really made it big." But he got way more out of it than expected when David Poor, a staffer at the Rock and Roll Hall of Fame, put him on the phone with Felix Cavalliere, the organist and lead singer of the '60s and '70s group the Rascals. As Dawson recalls it: "I was in the rehearsal room working with six other musicians, some of them just starters, and I wanted to teach them 'Good Lovin.' At the very end of that song is a wonderful trill, or flutter. I was playing it incorrectly and Dave taps me on the shoulder and says, 'How about if we give Felix a call?' I said, 'Sure, great.' Next thing I know he's handing me the phone and Felix Cavalliere talked me through how to play that note." The experience so energized Dawson that after camp he started his own moonlighting band and is having the time of his life—after the stock market closes. "It gave me an incredible boost in my musical self-esteem. This is the most fun I've had with my clothes on in years."

Several major league baseball teams, including the New York Mets, the Los Angeles Angels of Anaheim, and the Atlanta Braves have camps that allow you to play alongside baseball legends at spring training. Or for an all-inclusive fee you can join former Oriole great Cal Ripken Jr.'s fantasy camp in a four-day session in which you will receive instruction from Cal and several Oriole players. Baseball not your thing? Improve your tennis skills at the Chris Evert fantasy camp (www.evertacademy.com); learn how to drive a race car at the Richard Petty Driving Experience (www.1800bepetty.com); or become a weekend cowboy at the Sankey rodeo school (www.sankeyrodeo.com). You get the idea.

Meanwhile, technology is opening new doors to fun without leaving the house. If you're not online you're part of a rapidly shrinking demographic missing out on a wide range of leisure activities from the comfort of your own couch.

What's online? Everything! We don't have to tell you about

e-mail. Most people closely associate the Net with the ability to send electronic messages to friends and family anywhere in the world. But did you know that there are regional organizations almost everywhere, known as the free-net movement, dedicated to keeping Internet service affordable and promoting a free-flowing exchange of ideas on government and other matters of regional and national interest? If you want to exercise your activist muscles in your power years, one way to do it is by leading an online discussion of, say, the safety issues at a nearby nuclear power plant or the merits of a local proposed development. Or why not start your own Web log, known as a "blog," and report or opine on the Net on any subject you like? Thousands are doing it, and some are even getting famous.

Beyond e-mail, many Web surfers have discovered how to play bridge (www.okbridge.com) or backgammon (www.itsyour turn.com) or chess (www.chessclub.com) online. If you belong to AOL, these games are easily accessed and you can play against people anywhere in the world while holding a side chat with your opponent. In the area of games, nothing is hotter than gaming—casino-style gambling online. Internet gaming is now a $4 billion-a-year business and growing. An estimated eighteen hundred gambling sites have gone into business since 1995, virtually all of them operating in places such as Antigua, Costa Rica, and the Isle of Man.

A word of caution is appropriate here. While many folks find gambling in a casino to be relaxing, online gaming appears to be especially attractive to problem gamblers. The key missing ingredient at home—the thing that makes casinos fun—is the exotic and elaborate decor; the sound of the action, the drinks and food, and the company of other gamers. Without all that it's just betting, and not terribly fun unless you win, which of course nearly no one does on a long-term basis. The Gambling Treatment Center at the University of Connecticut found that 75 percent of those who regularly gamble online have a gambling problem, versus only 5 percent with a gambling problem from the total gambling population. That said, there are those who honestly enjoy and can handle and afford the action right at home. For roulette, craps, slots, and more, check out www.casinonnet.com or www.partypoker.com or www.30topcasinos.com. Before you get started you might check out what they say at www.gamblers anonymous.org or another help site, www.ncgambling.org.

For a different kind of Web fun, many adults have turned to tracing their ancestry. Roy Pilson of Staunton, Virginia, loves to scour the Net for genealogy records and to stay in touch via e-mail with the more than two hundred members of the Pilson Family Association. Using the Web, he's found access to all sorts of county and state records, and has gotten into libraries all over the country. "You can find something about just about anything you can think about," says Pilson. Some good starting points are www.ancestry.com, www.rootsweb.com, and www.ellisisland.org.

If tracing your past isn't your thing, you can use the Web to seek your future. Increasingly, America's adult singles are going online to find love. We'll get into Web dating in more detail in Chapter 3.

Sharing Good Times

Extended periods of leisure offer a great opportunity to enhance the relationships that matter most: family and close friends. You can use your newfound free time to strengthen bonds with the important people in your life, starting with your mate. When they were young, work often overwhelmed Norma and Maurice Joseph from Hampshire, England. Norma was a fashion director at the House of Worth, and Maurice owned a chain of restaurants. They had almost no time for each other, and felt they were slowly drifting apart. Seeking a balance, they down-sized their careers and refocused on their marriage, building a new and loving life around their greatest passion: travel and adventure.

Since turning sixty they have visited more than one hundred twenty countries. They have cruised the 1,336 miles of Burma's great Irrawaddy River, seen the minefields of Cambodia, traveled the frontier between Pakistan and China, dog-sledded in Québec, fed sharks in Tahiti, rafted down Ethiopia's Omo River, crewed a hundred-year-old ship through the Tonga islands, and discovered the Dalai Lama's old car when visiting Tibet. The Josephs are now more in love than ever and aren't slowing down. Says Norma, "I'll take your number and when I feel I'm too old, I'll let you know."

For Erma Marak, new adventures helped deepen her relationship with her grown daughter, Judy. The two backpacked along the Pacific Crest Trail from Mexico to Canada. "It was a religious retreat for us," Erma said. "We backpacked 2,638 miles, and it took 138 days. The trip brought us closer together for the rest of our lives." Later, the two tackled the John Muir Trail, which runs two hundred twenty miles from Yosemite across eleven mountain passes to Mount Whitney. The trips reinforced a healthy mutual respect between mother and daughter, and that respect helps them get through the occasional rough patches that develop with one another in their day-to-day lives.

Travel adventure helped Carol Madsen, sixty, get closer to her best friends. She organized a hiking trip to explore the El Camino de Santiago, a five hundred-mile pilgrimage trail honoring St. James the apostle in northwestern Spain. Combining her love of hiking and camaraderie, she formed her group called the Hiking Highs, consisting of middle-aged hiking enthusiasts. To help with logistics, she went to Spanish Steps (www.spanish steps.com), a tour group that provided a guide and a package of lodging and meals. The women started in the tiny village of Molinaseca and headed west toward the cathedral in Santiago, about fifty miles from the Atlantic coast. They spent nights in hundred-year-old country homes. "It's very green and the wild-flowers were gorgeous," Madsen said, adding that you "could walk for a couple of hours and maybe pass one or two people." Such time and quiet proved invaluable in exploring the interests and opinions of her friends, whom she came to think of as sisters.

If you're looking to deepen your relationships with grand-children, nieces, or nephews, Grandtravel (www.grandtrvl.com) will tailor a trip developed by teachers, psychologists, and leisure counselors to areas with natural attractions (glaciers, jungles, mountains, canyons), historical sites (native villages, ancient cities, medieval castles), and other cultural attractions. At Adventure Women (www.adventurewomen.com), the focus is on building relationships among women where at least one is older than thirty. Gwen Marelli, forty, and her sixty-eight-year-old mother, Evelyne Tannehill, took a weeklong Lewis & Clark canoe and camping trip, enjoying each other while exploring the Missouri River in Montana along with a historian who com-mented along the way. The trip was Gwen's mother's idea, seeing it as a way to break their routines and spend some special time together. The two live five hundred miles apart, Gwen in Rancho Palos Verdes, California, and her mother in Reno, Nevada.

"One of the moments I remember best was a rock-climbing hike we took one afternoon after we came off the river for the day," says Gwen. "The hike was pretty strenuous and we had been paddling for seven hours on the river, and only a couple of us decided to partake with the two guides. My mom was cer-tainly the oldest one to go. It was a tough hike but we had a great view of the whole river from up top. When we came back into camp, the rest of the group was sitting around ready for dinner and they all applauded my mom for her accomplishment. The roles were reversed. I was the one who was very proud of her. Our mother-daughter trip became more like very close girl-friends having time away from the 'boys' rather than the typical parent-child getaway."

Rediscover Yourself

Phil Hendrix, a retired teacher, recently took his twenty-eight-foot wooden sailboat for a two-year, six-thousand-mile journey from San Francisco through the Panama Canal to Fort Lauderdale, Florida. Asked why, he responds, "A better question is, 'Why not?'" Near the Mexico-Guatemala border, a whale breached alongside his boat during a raging storm. Hendrix remembers looking in the whale's eye. "It was like he was communicating. I don't know what, but something, and it wasn't malevolent. Then the rain stopped. The sea died down, the wind quit, and the sun came out. We dried out in fifteen minutes, just as we left Mexican waters and entered Guatemala's. You won't get that on an airplane ride from point A to point B," says Hendrix.

You can use your new leisure hours to discover things about yourself that had been buried beneath the baggage of decades of unrelenting devotion to family and career. Self-discovery, wherever we find it, is a wonderful thing. When we were young, everything we did resulted in a sense of discovery, either about ourselves or the world around us. Our new experiences helped us grow and define what we wanted to study in college and later do for a living, and the kind of person we ultimately wanted to become. We lived for our experiences and searched out new ones wherever we could. Our power years provide a perfect time to rediscover discovery. They can be a time for reinventing ourselves, for late blooming and new beginnings—a time to push beyond what we've already become to explore and grow into what we truly want to be.

Garth Fisher tackled the Appalachian trail, fulfilling a long-held goal. "At sixty, I was at a stage and place in my life where I could plan and do such a journey. . . . I took to the task with the question to myself, 'Can I do it?' I learned that the answer was 'Yes.' In the months since my return to my old life, a part of me has remained on the trail. . . . The Appalachian Trail gave many experiences to me. These experiences came in the form of personal introspection, spiritual insights, personal changes, and lessons such as learning to accept help and gifts from others." For more on the many benefits of hiking and how to get started, check out the American Hiking Society (www.americanhiking .org). In Europe, try www.sherpaexpeditions.com for hiking trips through England's beautifully rugged lake district or www .activity-ireland.com to check out trails in Ireland. Or you can go to www.puretrailsnewzealand.co.nz to plan an expedition through some of the most scenic real estate in the South Pacific.

At the heart of self-discovery is an imbued creativity that each of us possesses. Creativity is not just about writing songs or poetry or inventing a faster computer chip. Being open to new experiences and realizing that new experiences are the keys to self-discoveries that enhance your life is part of the creative spirit in all of us. It is always present no matter how little it is exercised, and it can change us for the better in our power years.

As we mature, we naturally acquire a key ingredient for creativity: life experience. Indeed, wisdom and creativity are closely intertwined. If nurtured and allowed to flourish, our creative spirit can enhance our power years in four important ways, according to Dr. Gene Cohen, director of the Center on Aging, Health, and Humanities at George Washington University, and author of *The Creative Age*. Creativity strengthens our resolve in the face of loss or defeat by making us "more emotionally resilient," Cohen argues, adding that "just as exercise improves our muscle tone, when we are creatively engaged our emotional tone is elevated." Creativity also contributes to physical health as we age, he argues, citing studies that show "that a positive outlook and sense of well-being have a beneficial effect on the functioning of our immune system and our overall health." Creativity adds depth to our relationships, adds Cohen, by making us more appreciative of our later years and willing and likely to stay connected to younger people. And Cohen reflects that creativity is perhaps our greatest legacy, achieved by providing the next generation with "an invaluable model of what is possible as we age."

Laurin McCracken of Memphis, Tennessee, was winding down his career as a marketing executive for an architectural firm at age sixty-one when he discovered a passion for painting. He found success quickly. His *White Roses* watercolor won the Dolores Rogers Memorial Award at the Niagara Frontier Watercolor Society National Exhibition, and now his paintings sell for $3,500 apiece and his work goes on display at major art exhibits throughout his region. "My business plan is this—take three trips a year for two to three weeks at a time to places like Tuscany; eat well, sketch, take photos, come back, and do enough watercolors that will pay for the next trip and that will allow me to write off the last trip."

Maybe painting isn't your thing. At age fifty-nine James Harding of Longview, Texas, joined a junior college theater group. Or how about Lou Tudor of San Diego, who at fifty-six joined the Late Bloomers Comedy Improv Troupe? The number of retiree-oriented performing groups in the United States has grown from seventy-eight in 1999 to more than four hundred today, according to Bonnie Vorenberg, author of *Senior Theater Connections*, which is a rich resource for aspiring thespians past age fifty-five. "I've always been too introverted to mix really well," Harding told *Time* magazine. "But when I read an article in the local paper about acting class for adults, I remembered acting in high school plays, and that had been a happy time for me." Harding is among thousands of adults who have gone into theater in recent years as an avenue of self-expression, therapy, social benefit, and sheer fun. Indeed, adult theater is blossoming around the world, from England's legendary Winchester Dramatic Society at the newly rehabbed nine-hundred-year-old Chesil Theatre to the Older Women's Network Theater Group in Blacktown, Australia.

According to Joy Reilly, associate professor of theater at Ohio State University, "Often people's first reaction to joining a theater group is, 'I'm too old to memorize lines.' And I tell them, 'You're never too old to memorize; it'll just take longer, and it's good for your brain.'" Then they get to it and are amazed at what they can still do, she says. Opportunities abound through community colleges such as the one Harding went to, Kilgore Junior College in Longview, and at state universities such as UNLV, or Ohio State in Columbus, Ohio, which hosted the first International Senior Theater Festival and Conference in the United States and is weighing offering a master's degree in adult theater.

To learn what's available in your community, check with local schools. Most states have an arts council or foundation. Many cities have an arts center, which can be a fountain of information for opportunities for self-expression and discovery that run the gamut from sculpting to cooking. You can also check out Older Adult Service Information System (www.oasisnet .org), a national nonprofit educational organization charged with helping people get the most out of life through programs in the arts, humanities, wellness, technology, and volunteer service; or the Flying Colors Art Workshops (www.flyingcolorsart.com), which allow you to study under artists around the world. In its Athens program you may visit and paint the island of Mykonos and explore the ancient civilization of Akrotiri. In its Ireland program you can paint the rugged beauty of the western regions and visit the Lisdoonvarna hot mineral baths or tour a castle on the secluded Aran island of Innisheer.

At Crow Canyon Archaeological Center (www.crowcanyon .org) you can work alongside professional archaeologists exploring ancient sites of the Pueblo Indians. If you have a culinary bent: at Dante Alighieri Siena Committee (www .dantealighieri.com) you can study Italian among the Italians, and with Pata Negra (www.patanegra.net) you may take exclusive cooking courses in Spain. La Varenne's (www.lavarenne.com) offers a five-day master cooking class in Burgundy, France.

The options are multiplying. In our power years we'll be able to tap the creativity we all possess to find our hidden passions and discover new ones, and continue to grow and blossom through the ageless process of self-discovery.

See, Feel, Taste, and Touch the World

Travel and adventure are deeply ingrained in the boomer psyche. Leaving our usual haunts and patterns puts us in front of new people, cultures, and experiences we'd never encounter at home. Dorothy Robinson of Stockton, California, travels ten times a year with Elderhostel (www.elderhostel.org) and Earthwatch (www.earthwatch.org). Her trips enable her to engage all kinds of people and cultures around the world. "I'm not about sitting around a hotel lobby," she sniffs. "I prefer no phone, no TV, no nothing. If I had to have those things, I wouldn't leave home. I don't want to see a hotel show with native costumes. I want to meet the people where they live."

During a trip to Lake Naivasha, Kenya, she helped determine which commercial fish could be introduced into the lake. "Instead of a hotel show, I sat by the water and watched fishermen clean their fish at dusk. They told us not to go into the water after dark because a croc comes up to eat the scraps. So that was our entertainment; we sat by the water watching a croc eat," Robinson said.

Although adventure and recreation are typically portrayed as provinces of the young, Ageless Explorers are increasingly becoming ones to push through long-standing boundaries. Lincoln Ellsworth was the first man to fly over both poles when he crossed Antarctica at age fifty-five. He discovered two uncharted mountain ranges and established the American Highland base on the little-known Indian Ocean coast. Hulda Crooks climbed eleven miles to the top of Mount Whitney, the highest peak in the continental United States, an amazing twenty-three times between ages sixty-six and ninety-three. At sixty-seven, Emma Gatewood became the first woman to solo-hike the twenty-one-hundred-mile Appalachian Trail. For an encore, she did it twice more. At fifty, Helen Thayer was the first woman to complete a solo ski trek all the way to the North Pole.

Several years ago, Age Wave put on a landmark conference on Healthy Aging attended by about a thousand health care executives. Helen Thayer was one of the speakers at the conference, and she arrived at the convention center just back from a jaunt to the North Pole. She was charming, gracious, and incredibly interesting. During the lunch break, Ken struck up a conversation with Dave Sliney, who was the head of marketing for Monsanto. Dave's flight had been late, so he missed the morning's sessions. Ken walked Dave over to Helen Thayer and introduced them. As they were walking away and Ken explained that Thayer had just hiked solo to the North Pole, Dave whispered back, "Now, why would anyone want to do that?"

Shortly after, Ken saw Helen in the hall, and when she asked him to tell her more about the gentleman she had just met, Ken responded, "He's head of marketing for Monsanto—a major global pharmaceutical and agribusiness firm." Thayer thought for a second and then leaned over to Ken and whispered in his ear, "Now, why would anyone want to do that?"

Some people like chocolate, others prefer vanilla. Some folks live to work, and others work to live.

The world awaits, and you'll find that more and more of tomorrow's adventurers will be men and women in their power years. Adventure vacations for people in their power years are among the fastest-growing travel segments.

Seeking to expand her horizons, Shige Kanei from Saitama Prefecture in Japan enrolled in an English-language school in

Los Angeles after leaving her job with the General Council of Trade Unions of Japan at age fifty-three. While in Los Angeles, her friends described the beauty and grandeur of South America, and at the first opportunity she put a few belongings in a backpack and headed south. She has spent most of her power years backpacking the world. She has been on every continent, stumbling across an annual festival in Tonga to taste traditional dishes such as spit-roasted pork with potatoes and fruit and witnessing eight-thousand-year-old rock drawings at Tassili. She travels on a tight budget, but because she has few time constraints she is able to get the cheapest plane tickets and take inexpensive local transportation. Frequently Kanei changes plans and takes off to a new country after hearing of an intriguing destination from fellow travelers. "Traveling offers a first for everything," she says. "It's full of surprises. That's why I can't stop."

Allen Young had always admired the Eco-Challenge Expedition Race, in which athletes travel a rugged three-hundred-mile course on mountain bike, river rafts, and horseback for one to two weeks. Intrigued by what has been called the world's toughest race, Allen traced the path of some of the world's best athletes—though at a leisurely pace—when he joined the Eco-Challenge Adventure Travel Program at age sixty-five. The program (www.ecochallengeat.com) allows you to visit remote locations where a recent race has taken place: British Columbia, Canada; Queensland, Australia; Morocco, North Africa; Patagonia, Argentina; Sabah, Malaysian Borneo; and the South Island of New Zealand.

Young's adventure expanded his vision of his own capabilities. "It was like an awakening that I could do this, and it was a great feeling," he says. "And everyone really pulled together to make it a great experience. I have memories that will last a lifetime. The new friends we made are a treasure. I learned much about what I could do."

There are lots of ways for you to experience the world. Check out Classical Cruises (www.classicalcruises.com) for a customized trip led by scholars and experts who will, for example, trace with you the journey of Odysseus in Homer's epic tale *The Odyssey*. This trip will take you to islands, caverns, and mountain peaks that are among the most stunning scenes in the Mediterranean. Nearly three-thousand years since Odysseus's mythical voyage, many of the sites identified with him still exist. The trip begins in Athens and continues to Troy; then to Lipari in the Aeolian Archipelago, long identified as the islands of Aeolus, the Lord of the Winds; to Malta, Calypso's domain; to Amalfi, the realm of the Sirens; and finally to Ithaca, Odysseus's long-sought home.

Fundación Sobrevivencia Cofan (www.cofan.org) will lead you through the ancient Zabalo rain forest in Ecuador guided by the Cofan people, the forest's original inhabitants. Andrew Johnstone of Chicago describes his trip as "simply amazing. I'd almost call it a transcendent experience, which sounds silly but is really the only way to describe it. We were essentially in the middle of totally pristine jungle. The sheer quantity and diversity of plant life is staggering."

With Asian Pacific Adventures (www.asianpacificadventures .com) you can travel to remote tribal festivals in Asia and be among the first foreigners to interact with natives. You can discuss Hindu philosophies with gurus at their ashrams, sit with Balinese masters in their home studios, share chai with Iranian scholars in a local teahouse, and dance with the village musicians in Vietnam. Or check out Myths and Mountains (www.mythsandmountains.com), which specializes in travel that gives you an inside view of cultures in the most exotic locations in Asia and South America. You will tour Bhutan with the son of the former king's courtier and be accompanied by a Buddhist monk through Tibet.

If active adventure in the great outdoors holds appeal for you, check out Canadian Voyageur Adventures (www.gocanoe .com), which provides guided excursions in replica fur-trade

canoes, or Knight Inlet Grizzly Bear Adventure Tours (www
.grizzlytours.com), which features grizzly bear viewing, whale
watching, rain forest hikes, and salmon fishing in British Columbia. Adventure Joseph Van Os Photo Safaris (www.photo
safaris.com) designs trips for nature shutterbugs in the world's
national parks, wildlife reserves, private ranches, tribal lands,
deserts, rain forests, remote islands, and wildlife migration
stopovers. Alpine Ascents (www.alpineascents.com) specializes
in global mountain climbs.

Just Do It!

Throughout most of your life you blocked out time for work and
your family's needs and squeezed in a little play around the
edges. Now you will increasingly be able to organize your time
however you like, putting leisure on an equal footing with work.
Strip away your old perceptions of recreation being largely a
way to relax and unwind. The new leisure can be spent testing
your limits and finding new interests, bonding with old friends,
and making new ones along the way. Putting leisure in this new
light will help you choose the experiences you'll want to try in
the years ahead. Instead of just being a break from work, you
will find that all the free time your power years will offer will
provide you with countless opportunities to truly liberate and
re-create yourself.

3

Rediscovering and Forging Vital Relationships

Whatever happened to the simple joy of sharing time with your spouse or a close friend? Your kids do it; they spend most of their free time hanging out with their pals, talking in the basement or out in the yard. There's no master planning out there. They aren't flapping on about college, grades, their likely career, or even what they want to do next summer. It's mostly playful prattle about other kids, a TV show or movie, or some silly observation such as green used to be their favorite color but now it's blue.

Kids with their friends. Isn't it great? But they aren't alone. Your parents probably do it, too; they have bridge clubs and investing clubs, and they golf with friends, shop, and go to long, schmoozy dinners in groups. They may hang out all afternoon with their group over lunch, chatting about their health or their grandkids, and making plans for tomorrow and next week.

During our hectic working and parenting years we programmed ourselves into believing that such idleness shows a lack of initiative and responsibility. Drinks or a long talk with a friend means taking time away from being productive. At the same time, though, most of us sense that we're giving up something valuable when we cut our hanging out time short.

You haven't been wrong to sacrifice friendships for career and family in your middlescence. You've probably had little choice. Blame it on soaring business travel, longer hours and more demands at work, and the flood of electronic infotainment that keeps you up to speed with just about everything you need—except other people. Many of us are so time-pressed that when we finally do get to dinner with other couples, everyone sets up their cell phones on the table like troops of U.S. Navy SEALS to be called into action on a moment's notice. And after an hour or so, members of the group usually peel off one by one to pick up the kids from baseball or soccer or dance or theater. For many, the combination of kids, needy parents, and demanding careers has squeezed out of life the nectar of unrushed relationship time.

In this chapter we'll explore rekindling the fires of your marriage, finding new love if you're single, and making new friends of all ages.

What are you giving up when you give up nurturing your key relationships? An awful lot, and maybe it's time to put our priorities in better order. Pick up any magazine devoted to success and you'll find that the only measure that seems to matter is money. Dan's first book was titled *Masters of the Universe: Winning Strategies of America's Greatest Deal Makers*. While writing the book in the late '90s, he recalls once being pressed on what exactly makes the subjects in his book so great. Looking for a short answer, he responded, "Collectively, they're worth about $10 billion." But the sharp questioner was unimpressed. "Big deal. That just means they're rich—not great."

It was a point well taken, and it illustrates the extent to which we have come to associate material things with success. Unfortunately, you don't make the cover of success-oriented magazines because you have ten great friends; you get there because you have $10 billion.

We're hopeful that our decades focusing on getting ahead will give way to simpler, more meaningful pleasures in our power years, as we'll again have the opportunity to rediscover the value of just sharing time with those we love. In the years ahead, your kids will leave home if they haven't yet and your job will become a secondary focal point. Not so suddenly, but perhaps surprisingly, you'll find that you have a huge opening in your life into which friendships can reemerge and be nurtured purely for the sake of having fun.

As good as that might sound, you may actually have to relearn how to make and develop meaningful relationships. Even if you remain happily married you might crave a new circle of friends, and the sad truth is that you may be woefully out of practice when it comes to creating and feeding those kinds of personal ties. As you've been busy building a family and making a living, friendships have been tossed aside, not for lack of interest but for lack of time and energy. Intimacy may have gone the same route.

New Yorkers Debra and Gary Kreissman got a firsthand lesson in what's expendable when time constraints mount. Frustrated with their flagging social life, they organized what they figured would be a simple proposition: three couples for a relaxed evening of reconnecting and wine-tasting at their apartment. Not once, but twice after they had firm commitments from the group, they ended up canceling the party at the last minute because several of their guests had to travel for business or family reasons. "A social event like this just isn't a priority anymore," says Gary.

Okay. You're strapped for time and a little out of practice. Will you really have to learn how to make friends, and even how to make love, all over? Isn't a lifetime of living all the education you'll need to understand even complicated relationships? In a word, no. Your lifetime of living may be precisely what has eroded your bonding skills. Now, as you ponder the looming opportunity to plug this yawning hole in your life, you may be mystified and not have anyone to whom you can turn. Thousands of books have been written about managing the financial aspects of life, but far too few are available on how to maintain, grow, or initiate love and friendship in adulthood.

For previous generations, creating new friendships or starting new relationships in adulthood wasn't as difficult to scope out or manage. Most people spent their lives in one community and didn't live long enough to have to worry about finding and nurturing late-life friends and lovers. And just a hundred years ago, several generations of a family typically lived under the same roof, on the same city block, or near the family farm. But in the twentieth century, career pursuits, lifestyle preferences, and just plain wanderlust caused families to become fanned out across the globe. In addition, folks started living so long that some marriages began to run out of steam at an age when people had routinely died.

Maybe the old model of having a best friend from cradle to grave or one spouse till death do you part will ultimately be retired along with the word "retirement." Anthropologist Margaret Mead was once asked to reflect on her failed unions. "I didn't have any," she argued. "I've been married three times and each marriage was successful." How could that be? Mead explained that over her many years, she had gone through several distinct stages as an adult. During each stage she had become in essence a different person with new likes and dislikes and in need of a different set of characteristics and priorities from her mate. She did not look back on her three marriages as failures because they didn't last, but rather as perfect partnerships for each different phase of her life.

We realize that late-life divorce can be especially hard on your other relationships. You can—and some do—break up at fifty and then move forward into decades of a new life, maybe even with more children. The result of this modern lifestyle is a challenging new dynamic: total strangers are introduced into the home with staccato regularity, often turning traditional age parameters inside out and greatly complicating our ability to enjoy an old-fashioned nuclear family.

Dan and his wife Kim confront this reality every holiday season. His parents are in their seventies. Her parents are divorced; her father is in his sixties, remarried to a woman with three sons in their twenties. Her mother is in her fifties and usually shows up with a boyfriend aged anywhere between thirty and seventy, with any number of teens in tow—and with one or two guest dogs to boot.

In this relatively small family, every decade since the 1930s is represented. No generation is quite sure what TV shows to watch as a group or what the other is talking about over dinner. The result is that many conversations are an abruptly starting and stopping stream of non sequiturs, and conversations often devolve into comic interrogation:

Grandma: "The darn plovers are mating again."

Teen: "Who are the Plovers?"

Grandma: "You know the plovers, sweetie. They live near me on the shore."

Teen: "I'm not sure I remember your neighbors, Mr. and Mrs. Plover. But you say they're having regular sex?"

Grandma: "I guess you could put it that way. All I know is that when they're mating I can't go to the beach."

Teen: "For gosh sakes, Grandma, why not? Are you too busy peeking in their window?"

Grandma: "What window? They're on the beach."

Teen: "Your neighbors like sex on the beach?"

Grandma: "No. My neighbors drink scotch, dear. The plovers are birds. Every year they nest in the dunes, and large sections of the oceanfront get roped off to keep the eggs safe. So when the plovers are mating I have to stay off the beach."

Teen: "I get it, Grandma. And as long as you have to stay off the beach you might as well sneak a peek of the neighbors going at it like a pair of barnyard animals, huh?"

Rekindling the Fires

Making sure that love flowers in adulthood requires commitment and energy. With your longtime spouse or partner you may need to bring some wattage back into the relationship to replace the energy that may have left home with the last child. How do you do that? It's been a long time since you had time to really focus on your mate. Now you can. Perform small acts of consideration, such as surprising her with flowers or buying him the CDs or DVDs he loves. Don't be afraid to be corny and sweet or to go out on dates. Even after many years together your spouse will appreciate the gestures.

Most important: talk over the need to reconnect. What should you do more of? What would you rather stop doing? Your spouse will be thrilled to hear how much you value the relationship and how committed you are to making it last. And don't be shy about reintroducing romance into your relationship. How do you do that?

Ken and his wife actually get remarried every year. Ken says:

When we originally married, on Thanksgiving in 1983, we had such a great time on our honeymoon that I asked Maddy if she'd consider remarrying me every year—but in a different religion and in a different location each Thanksgiving.

We haven't missed a year yet, and so far, we've been remarried in a castle in Bath, England, by an Anglican priest, in a Hopi ceremony in Sedona, Arizona, in a Navajo ceremony in Tucson, Arizona. We've been married while skiing in Vail, while nude in a Tai Chi ceremony at Esalen Institute in Big Sur, California, and while on a boat in the Sea of Cambodia off the coast of Thailand. We've recited our vows in Grace Church in Greenwich Village, in a Buddhist ceremony in Berkeley, California, in a Mayan wedding at the top of the Chichan Itza pyramid in the Yucatán, and, of course, at the Chapel of Love in Las Vegas. We've even been "married" by our children on a beach in Mexico. In fact, we also had our kids perform the ceremony when we celebrated my parents' sixtieth anniversary by staging a formal remarriage ceremony and party. When my dad strolled down the aisle in his white dinner jacket arm in arm with my beaming mom and then our kids launched into their service, it was an incredibly powerful moment in all of our lives— for every reason you can think of.

Getting remarried each year is a lot of fun. But we also have found that these occasions are valuable moments when we can look critically at the year that just passed and openly discuss what went wrong and what went right. We also have practical discussions of what our relationship needs more of or less of. This annual ritual has proven a great way for us to stay connected even while our kids are at home; it has helped us remember the things that made us fall in love in the first place and allows us to take notice of all the reasons we love each other still.

Different couples honor and rediscover their love in different ways. After retiring from dual high-powered careers, Edrie and Tony Shenuski of Scottsdale, Arizona, grew closer by taking a cooking class at the Scottsdale culinary school. Both of them grew up in households with fond memories of their parents spending many fun hours in the kitchen. But Edrie, a former pharmaceutical industry executive, and Tony, a former IBM and

America Online executive, didn't have time to replicate that experience in two decades of marriage with two kids and, later, two grandkids. Now in their power years they can't wait to whip up new concoctions together in their custom two-chef kitchen. "I always appreciated good food but never really cooked because I worked long hours and traveled so much," Tony says. Adds Edrie: "Cooking together has been a great way to connect. I think cooking brings couples together." She has a point. Corning Ware recently surveyed married and engaged couples and found a kitchen love link: 82 percent of couples who cook together at least a few times a week reported being very satisfied with their relationships compared to only 73 percent of those who seldom cook together.

Cooking, of course, is just one pastime that might help you grow closer to your spouse. Feel free to substitute any activity (old or new) that the two of you might enjoy—hiking, cycling, running marathons, playing golf, spinning clay, throwing paint at a canvas, traveling, or volunteering at a soup kitchen. Staying busy at something each of you enjoys can help you rediscover the character traits and common interests that initially ignited your passion for one another decades ago. This kind of rediscovery may be all that stands between your loving union and a decline into what psychotherapist Douglas LaBier, director for the Center for Adult Development in Washington, D.C., calls a "functional relationship." That's a marriage where the spark has disappeared but the relationship still works somewhat because it's centered on practical concerns like who takes out the garbage or brings the car in for repair. Functional marriages may last until death because for both husband and wife there's at least some comfort in having a reliable partner to help you deal with life's logistical challenges.

If you want romance, passion, and spark in your marriage, you can get it, but you'll have to do more than be Johnny-on-the-spot with dinner or send out the Christmas cards on time. You'll have to keep growing and remain interesting to the one who knows you best. In your power years you'll be able to re-explore the interests that first attracted your spouse as well as many new ones, and keep the old flames flickering.

Equally important, though, is that you do not suffocate one another. The ability to spend more time together is a blessing that can quickly become a nightmare if you expect your spouse to share all of your interests, or if you want to spend so much time with your spouse that he or she cannot pursue separate interests that hold little appeal to you. In other words, you need some alone time, and it's important that in your alone time you pursue activities that help you grow as an individual and remain an interesting person with new insights and surprising responses. Your spouse was not attracted to you in the beginning because he or she knew everything about you and loved it all. Your spouse was attracted partly by the mystery that you presented, and the more he or she learned, the stronger your bond grew. It's critical that you keep growing on your own and keep giving your spouse more to find out. Book clubs and investment clubs are great ways to learn and become more interesting. So is any kind of artistic pursuit or continuing education or volunteer activity. Now that your relationship has matured, don't get lazy. You both lose if you do.

Finding New Love

One day early in Ken's career, he found himself visiting the vast Sun City retirement complex in Arizona as part of his research on aging. Ken recalls,

In the evening, as I was checking into a motel across the street, I was struck by a dull thumping sound that was pulsating through the walls around me and literally shaking the floor beneath my feet. Curious, I followed the beat down a hallway beyond the lobby and into a large but dimly lighted motel lounge, where a DJ was spinning music from *Saturday Night Fever*. John Travolta was nowhere in view. But the joint was rocking, jammed tight with women in layers of makeup and snugged into short skirts and low-cut blouses; the men wore open shirts with gold chains draped around their necks.

It was the '70s, and anyone would have recognized this scene as a singles meat market. What made it so striking, though, was that no one in the room was a day under seventy. I was at first incredulous, then amused. These were grandmas and grandpas. Didn't these folks see how zany they looked? Yet after surveying the room for a little while I reconsidered. What makes anyone think that mature singles aren't or shouldn't be on the make? They clearly were trolling for action here at the Thunderbird Inn some thirty years ago. And guess what? They are today, too—and with more vigor than you might suppose. The libido doesn't fail us at sixty or seventy or even eighty. If Bob Dole was able to go on TV and sell Viagra by the bucketful that should be all the evidence you need.

Many of us will be blessed with long, happy marriages that provide both friendship and intimacy. Neither Ken nor Dan can envision life without their first and only wives. But the reality is that many people will divorce at a relatively early age, and many more will become single through the death of a spouse. In times past, little thought was given to finding a new soulmate if these life events occurred past age sixty. But with longer lifetimes today that leaves another thirty or so years to explore a whole new love, and you should not let those years slip by.

Ken tells this story about his mother-in-law, Sally:

In the late 1980s, my wife's father died of cancer at a youthful age sixty. My mother-in-law, Sally, found herself a widow at fifty-nine after having been with the same man since high school. It was a sad time. Sally felt as though she had been cast adrift as she tried to sort out what she would do with the rest of her life. One year after she had been widowed, Sally called and said she wanted to talk about something that was "troubling her." I worried that she might be grappling with a personal crisis or illness; she had asked that I come alone. So I flew to Los Angeles the next day and met her in a quiet restaurant.

We sat down. She suggested I have a glass of wine. "No thanks, not tonight," I said. "What's wrong?" Feeling nervous, Sally repeated her offer to pour me a glass from the bottle of Merlot she had ordered. I declined again, and asked what was going on.

Sally took a deep breath. "Ken, I need to talk with someone about sex," she started. "Since I trust you, I'm hoping you can help me make sense of something that's really got me hung up." I quickly decided some wine might not be such a terrible idea after all, and downed a glass. "What do you mean?" I asked.

"Well, you know, I'm sixty-one. I'm still a somewhat attractive lady. Men are starting to ask me out. I may be alive twenty or thirty more years and I'll probably find myself dating at some point, and I'll be honest with you, I've never dated. I've never been with another man, and I missed the whole sexual revolution. I'd like for you to fill me in."

I helped myself to another glass of wine. "Oh, you mean you want to know the trends and social dynamics of the sexual revolution?"

"No," she said, "I want to know the real practical,

personal stuff. How many times does a guy expect you to date him before you put out, and at whose apartment? And who's on top? Who's on bottom?"

I was now ordering another bottle, but also wondering: just where does a fifty- or sixty-plus woman go to talk about sexuality? There aren't many books on the subject, and there aren't many segments about sex and the single grandma on morning TV. So I took the deep dive and began to discuss with Sally all I know about adult sexuality. When dinner ended three hours later, I hugged my mother-in-law and headed back to the airport. During the next year, the topic didn't come up again. But as Sally began to date various suitors, I wondered if she was taking my advice.

A few months later Sally called and, with both Maddy and me on the phone, she breathlessly announced, "I'm in love."

"You can't be in love Mom," Maddy insisted. "You're still on the rebound, and you don't know what love is anymore."

"No," she said, "I'm really in love, and with a fabulous man."

"Gee, when did you meet this guy?" Maddy inquired.

"Two days ago," Sally responded.

There was a long silence as Maddy and I wondered if Sally had gone a little nuts. But the story got even better, because Sally then said, "And I'd like for you to come meet him as soon as possible, because we're thinking about getting married."

"Where does he live?" Maddy asked.

"Here."

"Oh, he's a neighbor?"

"No," Sally gushed, "he lives right here with me. He moved in this morning. Isn't that great?"

Maddy and I feared the worst, that the stress of being alone had driven Sally crazy or that she was being taken advantage of. But the following month we met Sally's new beau, Ray, and quickly came to understand that the two were truly in love. They were holding hands, and laughing, and sharing their dreams for the years ahead. Sally and Ray were bubbling with excitement about the trips they would take, the courses they would sign up for, and the things they would do together.

That was all ten years ago, and since then their love for one another has grown beyond even their expectations. They have truly crafted a new life for themselves, different and just as good as what they had experienced with their previous mates. And our entire family has come to love and admire Ray—he's a terrific man, a wonderful stepdad, and a loving grandfather to our children.

Part of living longer is having sexual desire longer—for both sexes—and potent drugs such as Viagra, Levitra, and Cialis are hardly the only wonders of modern medical science turning up the heat. Have you seen Goldie Hawn or Heather Locklear lately? A healthy lifestyle combined with a youthful attitude (and for some perhaps a touch of cosmetic surgery) can keep both men and women sexy well past the day when we always assumed Mom and Dad had put away the sex toys.

This isn't an easy subject for a lot of people. Sex beyond the procreating years has long been a taboo area of discussion, reflected in the pejorative words and phrases we commonly use when addressing the issue. "Our language is full of telltale phrases: older men become 'dirty old men,' 'old fools,' or 'old goats' where sex is involved," write Drs. Robert Butler and Myrna Lewis in *The New Love and Sex After Sixty*. "An older woman who shows an evident, perhaps even a lusty interest in sex is assumed to be suffering from emotional problems; and if she is obviously in her right mind and sexually active she runs the risk of being called oversexed. What is perceived as lustiness in young men is often seen as lechery in older men."

These harmful misconceptions are deeply ingrained. But they are starting to wear down as our generation—famous for being loose with love—advances and promises to be on the make right up to the very limits of life.

The good news, assert Drs. Butler and Lewis, is that the physical changes our bodies go through as we age appear to have very little impact on our ability to engage in sex into our eighties, especially with performance-enhancing drugs. Pharmaceutical companies are now feverishly developing drugs that will promote sexual response in women, and these should be on the market in the very near future.

Is sex for life the most important ingredient in adult relationships? We don't think so. Most people are more worried about not having someone to talk to and to do things with, such as go to the movies or out to dinner. Even at younger ages, sexual desires range a great deal. You may not require or even want an active sex life in your power years. There's nothing wrong with that. But if you do, fulfillment will play an important role in maintaining your self-esteem. Our view of sexuality is changing. Consider the 2003 film *Something's Gotta Give* in which Jack Nicholson's character, who at sixty-two boasted of never having had sex with a woman over thirty, falls for the mother of one of his dates, the fiftysomething beauty played boldly by Diane Keaton. That's a sharp turn from the stereotypical adult male being attracted to a young girl that is so often depicted on film and TV.

If you're starting over because of divorce or death, the first question you might chew on is whether you even want to be married. Late-life marriages can have complications, from prenuptial agreements to obnoxious grown children. But there are good reasons to tie the knot: laws vary from state to state, but in general, husbands and wives can make medical decisions for one another, while unmarried partners cannot. And for what it's worth, your spouse cannot be forced to testify against you in court. Your grown kids may object to you remarrying, for reasons that may have to do with inheritance. If you're still catering to their wishes at this point in life you've got bigger problems than we can solve. Cut that cord and do what's right for yourself.

The good news for men is that they will be in demand: there are ninety-two men for every hundred women between ages fifty-five and sixty-five; and fewer men in every age group older than that. This can lead to a tough game of demographic musical chairs for women, who not only live longer than men by six or seven years but who also often get shut out of dates with their peer group because many men tend to prefer younger women.

In a poignant moment in the final season of the HBO series *Sex and the City*, Candace Bergen played a successful, single fiftysomething businesswoman. She fell for a fiftysomething character played by Mikhail Baryshnikov. But Baryshnikov's character happened to be in a relationship with the much younger Carrie, played by Sarah Jessica Parker. At the telling moment, Bergen's character sadly confronts Carrie and tells her it isn't fair that she steal from an older pool of eligible men.

We accept older men with younger women. Michael Douglas marrying Catherine Zeta-Jones and fathering a child? No big deal. But with the superior longevity of women and their greater likelihood of being left single and healthy, we'll have to get over our collective reluctance to accept the union of an older woman with a younger man. Who didn't regard Ashton Kutcher as Demi Moore's boy toy? But guess what? In an AARP survey of singles between ages forty and sixty-nine, one in three women said they had dated a younger man; 14 percent of women in their fifties said they prefer to date men in their forties or younger.

Spend an evening in the ritzy parts of Palm Beach and you'll likely be amazed at what you see: hundreds of extremely wealthy older women going to dinners and social functions with paid male escorts in their twenties. Why not? Rich men have been doing it for years, and this is clearly one way that mature women can get the attention they desire. Alas, paid escorts may never be a permanent solution. But some creative forces are taking shape now that will lessen the strain on women.

Getting Started in the Singles World

If you're just getting started looking for love, don't panic. The grown-up dating game has never been more interesting. Of the 105 million North Americans who are forty-five or older, nearly 40 percent—some thirty-six million—are currently single, according to the U.S. Census Bureau. The stigma of dating at fifty or sixty is fading, and even in the seventies and beyond the singles scene is much more widely embraced than was the case when Ken first chanced on the pulsating floors of Sun City's Thunderbird Inn years ago.

How will you find new love? Millions of men and women have already exploited personal ads, dating services, and Club Med–inspired singles vacations to pursue their amorous side. To jump-start your search, here are few places and approaches to consider:

Friends and family. An amazing thing happens when you let those around you know you're back in the game. For whatever reason, people (including your own kids, in some cases) love to play matchmaker. The introductions will start coming quickly, and you may find yourself meeting people without even knowing it was a setup. That happened with Carl and Mary Ann. Her grown son, Brian, surreptitiously arranged for the two to meet at a wedding, and he later pushed his mother to invite Carl to dinner. The two divorcees hit it off and later were married. "I wasn't aware that he was sizing me up" when we first met, Carl reflects of his first meeting with Brian. "But now I thank him."

Churches and synagogues. One of the most traditional ways for adult singles to meet is still one of the most effective, especially if faith plays an important role in your life. At church and other religious functions, you can meet people with shared values. And most large congregations host singles events. Laurencetta Watson, fifty-eight, had been a widow for nine years when she joined the singles ministry of Windsor Village United Methodist Church in Houston. She was just looking for someone to share time with. But at the first meeting she met her soulmate, Andrew Watson. Both were on their way to a card game. He won her heart by racing ahead without her knowing it, and when she arrived "he was there holding the door open for me."

The Internet. An AARP survey found that one in fourteen singles between ages forty and fifty-nine regularly uses the Internet to find dates, and of those over fifty-five in the survey, 43 percent said it's possible to meet via the Net and fall in love. The largest Web site in this game is www.match.com, boasting 1.5 million members over fifty, which is its fastest-growing segment. Right behind match.com are Yahoo! personals and eharmony.com. Both sites walk you through the process, from filling out your self-description to e-mailing prospective dates. Outside the United States, try www.datefloor.com in Canada, and www.loveaccess.com and www.foreigndatefinder.com to hook up anywhere in the world. If a mate with the same faith is important, type in, for example, "singles Catholic." You'll be directed to www.catholicsingles.com and www.catholicmatch.com. Type "Jewish" instead of Catholic and you'll get www.jdate.com and www.jmatch.com. Love basketball? "Singles basketball" turns up www.fitness-singles.com. Want to go dancing? Adding "dancing" turns up www.singlesonthego.com. Are you an environmentalist? Try www.greensingles.com. If you want to meet a brainiac, www.rightstuffdating.com joins singles with elite college degrees. Don't be shy. Tens of millions log on to dating Web sites each year, and while we have no idea how many of them find love, we're sure they do better than folks who aren't willing to take a chance.

Speed dating. This is a fairly new strategy and most familiar to young adults. At a bar or restaurant, an organized group of singles arrive and spend five to ten minutes each with five to ten "dates." Afterward the singles share feedback with the organizer, who matches those singles who have the most in common. For example, at www.8minutedating.com, singles are organized into groups of 25 to 35, 30 to 40, 35 to 45, and 45 to 60. Tom Jaffee, CEO and founder, comments, "A lot of over-forty guys just don't get it," he says. "They'll go to the same bar every night for eighteen years and not get a date, but for some reason they won't try speed dating." That is sure to change in coming years, Jaffee says. "We're going to find ways to reach this group with our marketing message. This is the way women want to meet men. It's social, it's safe, it's comfortable."

How does it work? Jaffee's company organizes and hosts dating events for single men and women in virtually every large city in the United States as well as locations in Canada, Australia, China, South Africa, Great Britain, and other nations. The "dates" sit down one-on-one eight times for eight minutes each in the course of an evening. The cost is $35. At the end of the night each participant indicates to the event sponsor who they would like to have a follow-up date with, and the sponsor then informs all of those who have found a match. Most people enjoy the experience, Jaffee says, adding that 90 percent ask for a follow-up date and 60 percent of those get one. "My goal is to make dating comfortable—not an ego-damaging experience," says Jaffee. To get started, check out his Web site or another, www.pre-dating.com.

Don't give up on finding love. What you may need to give up, though, is common misbehavior that gets in the way. A few sins to be avoided are: get over past relationships, give up trying to be perfect, let go of protecting yourself from hurt, and lose the Don Juan routine.

Making New Friends

In our power years we will rediscover the fun, pleasure, and comfort that comes with spending quality time with friends. We are going to reconnect with old friends and make new ones like no generation before us, asserts Dr. Jan Yager, a sociologist and author of *Friendshifts: The Power of Friendship and How It Shapes Our Lives.* "Because so many boomers either married late or divorced early many have had years of being single as adults, where friendships were the key relationships in their lives," Yager says. "For boomers, adult friendships have had a different emphasis than for generations where couples married young and stayed married for forty or fifty years." We innately understand the importance of friendship networks, even if we have not had the time to nurture them in our busy primary career and child-raising years, Yager asserts.

In our power years we'll find the time.

We know that children who have friends do better in school and that adolescents who are loners are far more likely to have psychological and social problems downstream. But having friends isn't just good for your mental state; it promotes physiological benefits, too, such as longer life and greater health. A study in the *Journal of the American College of Cardiology* concluded that women with strong social networks live less stressful lives and have a healthier heart. Men, too, appear less vulnerable to heart disease if they have a network of friends. Medical researchers have found that those with friends are more likely to survive major surgery and are even less likely to get cancer.

Having friends also makes you resilient. You are less afraid to express grief and fear, which can help you bounce back quicker from problems or crises. Even something as simple as a pen pal can help. An extensive study of northern California residents found that having ties to at least one close friend extends life. Another study, of 257 human resource managers, found that adults who have friends at work report not only greater productivity but also far higher workplace satisfaction.

It's likely that women will take the lead in the mature friendship revolution as we begin to say good-bye to the Noah's Ark style of living more appropriate to our younger and procreative years. Throughout the first two ages of man, there was always one boy for every girl, and nearly all of life's activities were oriented around heterosexual couples. With the coming of the Age Wave, there simply won't be enough men to go around. This is less of an issue for same-sex partners because their longevity rates are rising together. But millions of heterosexual women are discovering that it can be as nourishing to share life's ups and downs with a network of close friends as with one spouse. A trip to any geographic area with a high concentration of retirees will reveal the emergence of silver-haired Amazonian tribes—energetic and attractive groups of older women who go to the movies together, enjoy investing together, and who care for each other should a health problem arise. We believe that increasing numbers of boomer women will choose to live together with their friends in their power years—recapturing some of the communal spirit of their youth and blending it with the emotional and financial practicalities of their current lives.

The latest research shows that men also crave time to break free of the rat race and sit around with friends, kick a soccer ball with their children or grandchildren, or take a slow hike. After being on the battlefield for decades, many are coming to realize the madness of their patterns and simply want to smell the roses in their third age.

How do you make friends as an adult? Getting involved in a new hobby or career or anything that you truly enjoy is a simple way to remain attractive to others, to be open to new encounters and interesting to the family and friends with whom you socialize. Stimulating new pursuits give you an immediate way to connect with new people and sharpen your interpersonal skills. The rest—turning casual acquaintances into close friends, possibly lovers, and then tending to these new relationships—is entirely up to you.

Jan grew depressed after she and her husband relocated to Scottsdale, Arizona. Her husband was still at work and frequently traveled; she was left alone in an empty house with no family or friends. "It seems like everyone is from somewhere else," she complained. After a year of agonizing over her situation, she found out about the Scottsdale Newcomers Club, which was once a Welcome Wagon group but had transformed over the years into a full-fledged community organization of eight hundred women looking for new friends. And you don't even have to be new in town to belong. Now Jan has all the camaraderie she desires, hiking, shopping, playing bridge, going to lunch, and sharing books.

There are countless other options for meeting new friends, such as volunteer work for the parks department or a religious group, or community-based adult education programs. Remember, if you keep doing what you're doing now, and in the same way, you won't meet new people. Perhaps it's time to change some patterns and see what turns up. In seeking out new friends, try to work through two or more separate social networks.

People often get hung up on the notion of a best friend—one person who can fulfill every aspect of a relationship. But we don't have to have a single best friend; we can have a network of friends who fill different needs in our life. Some people will be great jogging or golfing partners while others will be better at traveling or discussing personal problems. In adulthood, men and women often find satisfaction in being able to express different parts of their personality with different kinds of people. It's healthy and it can provide a wide range of comforts and a broader social network to replace the contacts from work or family that may have diminished over the years.

Yager has found that shared values between friends such as honesty, fidelity, loyalty, fitness, or a sense of adventure are the best predictors of long-lasting friendships. Two people need not have identical likes and dislikes to become friends, but it helps if they share some core values. And it takes time. "I found that on average becoming a tried and true friend takes three full years," Yager says. "So take your time when you decide to get to know someone. Going slowly will help you avoid being disappointed because you too quickly trusted someone that you didn't really know."

Where can you hunt for new friends in your power years?

The office. Coworkers have a lot of common ground and can make wonderful friends. Bonds at work can extend into after-hours friendships as well.

Participants in educational courses or workshops. This is one of the best ways to meet new people and a great alternative to bars and singles clubs.

Churches, synagogues, or charitable programs. When people come together to do good things, pretenses and defenses are often down and the real person shines through. And if you're nervous about how to handle one-on-one encounters as you're getting your sea legs, these groups can be ideal for meeting terrific people and expanding your network.

People in your daily routine. This could be your next-door neighbor, one of your children's parents, or a fellow member of a civic, charitable, or activist organization. Getting to know on a somewhat more personal level people you see all the time can offer a sense of well-being and possibly blossom into something bigger.

People with similar interests. A jogging pal, shopping companion, book club or bridge partner can provide a social aspect to your favorite pastimes.

Friends from your past. People you went to college or grew up with or used to work with early in your career hold many common experiences that can be a strong foundation for a lasting relationship. If you get a chance to reconnect with an old friend, take it because a whole new phase of your friendship may follow.

The Internet. It's not just a way to meet eligible singles. You can meet friends there, too. Of course, many folks are prone to exaggeration when afforded the anonymity of a screen name. Even if the friendship never moves offline, these kinds of relationships can fill pockets of need and prove to be fun and rewarding.

While building new friendships in adulthood, experts suggest that you allow "friendshifts" to take place at their own pace. Moving a friendship to a higher level of intensity or frequency can be exciting, even exhilarating; letting a friendship fade away does not diminish what the relationship once gave you. Moving on is part of life, Yager points out. It comes with some risks. Your new friend may not be interested in stepping up the relationship. Most of the time they are. People crave connections and will usually be open to new ones with potential to become special. Meanwhile, if you're feeling that a friendship has grown stale and cannot be salvaged, the other person may feel it, too. Sometimes the best thing to do is move on.

Cross-generational Connections

Among the things you may have lost sight of over the past half century is the importance of ties between young and old, not just within your family but also throughout your community. We have become an age-segregated society. The kids go to school all day and have carefully orchestrated extracurricular activities through the dinner hour, all with their peers. Mom and Dad spend ever longer hours at the office with no children or elders in sight. Older adults live in retirement villages or congregate in senior centers with people their age. It's exacerbated by our spread-out extended families, which only occasionally come together. When they do, family members sometimes find they have virtually no common touchstones.

The result is that the old have too few relationships with the young; the young do not understand their elders or the aging process. This relatively new development has consequences well beyond our inability to relate in a meaningful way with those who are dear to us. In the absence of understanding, myths and stereotypes flourish. Young and middle-aged people see elders as feeble and intransigent. Elders see younger generations as disrespectful punks to be feared, not embraced. Potentially wonderful intergenerational relationships don't happen as they should.

A few years ago, the noted author and Harvard Law School professor Alan Dershowitz was at dinner with a group including his eight-year-old grandson, Lyle. At one point he turned to the boy and said he'd like to talk for a few minutes about school, to which Lyle shot back: "I'm sorry, but you're too boring to talk to. I just want to eat." Boring? In his career Dershowitz has held rapt some of the nation's brightest students, not to mention the legal and media elite. That was of no consequence to his grandson, however. To Lyle, Grandpa had become a snooze.

What could he do about it? This was no small matter. Like most grandparents, Dershowitz prizes his relationship with his children's children. Was it really possible that he and Lyle had lost the ability to connect? Sure. It happens all the time in today's far-flung families, where kids spend almost all of their time with peers instead of interacting with older and younger cousins, aunts, uncles, and grandparents. Happily for Dershowitz, though, the disconnection lasted but a moment. He was back in the game after quickly changing the subject to something little Lyle cared about: Spiderman.

To cement this small victory, Dershowitz agreed to allow Lyle and his only other grandchild, Laurie, ten, to begin calling him "Poppa Al." No big deal, you say? To Dershowitz it was. He cringes at the thought of the pizza shop moniker, and he has long despised being called Al by anyone. But in this case, it was simply worth it.

Intergenerational ties can keep your life interesting and connected while providing enormous emotional nourishment. Nearly twenty years ago Karen Glimmerveen took the first of many trips with her husband's mother, Jeanette Glimmerveen. "We love our trips," says Karen. "Our first ones were physically adventurous, canoeing the Green River and camping out, sailing the cape, hiking through the jungle in Belize. Just getting through one of those trips left us with a great feeling of accomplishment, and we enjoyed many laughs of the you-had-to-be-there variety." As the years went by, they scaled back the strenuousness of their journeys so that Jeanette could continue taking part. They called and faxed one another frequently while planning a trip, enjoying that give and take almost as much as the actual travel. On the road, they roomed together. "We found we are a little like sisters," says Karen. "Experiencing these many travels together has brought us very close; we have common stories to tell and pictures to share, jokes and wild experiences that no one else can understand. We genuinely like each other, and it's great to have my mother-in-law as a special friend."

Even if you're separated from family, you can create bonds outside of your age group by focusing on interests such as theater, poetry, fitness, dance, or astronomy, or by mingling with people of all ages who are neighbors or part of civic groups. Our innate desire as human beings to interact with people of varying ages may have taken a hiatus in the past half century, but it is reemerging today as our parents grow disenchanted with their isolation and we ponder the mistakes that led them there.

This quiet yen to stay connected outside your peer group may be one reason for the runaway success of a book such as *Tuesdays with Morrie* by Mitch Albom, which struck a nerve that had been dormant for too long. In this heartwarming real-life tale, Albom tells of reconnecting with a favorite college professor he hadn't seen in sixteen years. After learning his old mentor was dying of Lou Gehrig's disease, Albom visits the man every Tuesday and soaks up his wisdom on love, work, marriage, envy, children, forgiveness, community, and aging—all seen through the eyes of a man down to his last days on Earth.

Only one in three of today's grandparents are regularly and actively involved in the lives of their grandchildren, asserts Don Schmitz, author of *The New Face of Grandparenting*. That's partly because two in three grandparents have grandchildren who live more than a day's drive away. We believe that connecting with grandchildren can be of such value to you that it's important to find ways to be involved.

As we mature we more fully embrace the notion that relationships are what's important, and we discover that the third age of life provides both the time and the wisdom with which to build and harvest meaningful connections. A simple Christmas tradition—baking a fruitcake—changed the course of Faye and Trillie Brown's lives. The two sisters from Moundville, Alabama, today in their sixties, have collaborated on five books about growing up hearing about the Great Depression. They have no direct memory of those dark years. But every Christmas for as long as they can remember, their mother would gather all the children and grandchildren in the family and while sifting flour and greasing pans regale them with tales of daily life in the 1930s. It ignited a passion for that era that her daughters hang on to even now, as they bake fruitcakes every Christmas with every child and grandchild of theirs lucky enough to live nearby.

During Ken's annual week-long rafting trip with his son, Zak, they have noticed that each year the trips become increasingly populated by youthful and active grandparents taking the adventure with one or two of their grandchildren. The same thing is happening on cruises and safaris and all manner of trips and vacations. A transformation is under way: instead of playing checkers on the front stoop, we're shooshing down the slopes at Vail and hiking the Smokey Mountains and attending an Outkast concert with our grandchildren. Indeed, the single biggest driver getting folks over sixty-five online is their desire to e-mail distant grandchildren.

Make It Happen

How can you go about connecting with other generations? Not much will happen if you don't set things in motion. Compared to your own grandparents, you're probably a lot healthier, more mobile, and open to doing all sorts of things. Here are a few ways to make the most of your children, and their children.

Off to camp. One of the best ways to get quality time with grandchildren is to splurge on a getaway. Leave Mom and Dad behind. They'll thank you for it. The granddaddy of intergenerational camps is Grandparents' and Grandchildren's Camp (www .sagamore.org) at Great Camp Sagamore in Raquette Lake, New York, opened by famed family psychiatrist Dr. Arthur Kornhaber in 1986. His philosophy: time together in an idyllic setting without parental interference is the perfect backdrop for building a lasting relationship between grandparents and grandchildren. Don't worry about them misbehaving. Kids tend to be on their best behavior when Mom and Dad aren't around and they feel a huge sense of security when they know that someone other than their parents is there for them.

Many camps now cater to bookend generations. Bill Abler,

fifty-nine, found his answer at Grandkids and Me camp (www
.grandkidsandme.com) in Amery, Wisconsin, where up to thirty
campers bunk in dorm rooms overlooking Lake Icaghowan. He
spent a week there hiking, canoeing, building birdhouses, and
just talking with his granddaughter, Sadie, seven. "Now when I
go visit she hugs me, and then often we'll sit and talk or read a
book together," Abler recounts. "We're building a wonderful
bond." A weekend away is a natural way to dispel stereotypes
about Grandma and Grandpa as being sweet but no fun. When
kids see their elders hiking, water skiing, or doing anything that
requires energy and vitality, it opens up countless new doors
because they no longer see you as someone who needs to be
cared for but as a potential cool new friend—and one who will
spoil them to boot!

Elderhostel also has a variety of international programs,
including Canada, Europe, and Asia, for bookend generations
(www.elderhostel.org). Among their most popular events is
whale watching off the coast of Québec. You can find other
camps by going to Google and entering the term "grandparent-
grandchild camps." Among the leaders in organized "grandtrip-
ping" around the world are Grandtravel (www.grandtrvl.com),
and Thomson Family Adventures (www.familyadventures.com),
which plans trips from Turkey and Belize to Peru, China, and
Egypt.

Keep it fun. Okay, it took twenty-five years for your kids to gain
their independence and for you to gain your freedom. Odds are
they don't want you to move in with them, and even if they do,
you have no such inclination. That's understandable. But you
will always be welcome for frequent visits if you follow two simple rules: be helpful and don't be obnoxious. The last thing your
children need with their own children running amok in the medicine cabinet and playing on the stairs is another needy—or
bossy—person in the house. Grandparents who truly want to be

welcome in the home of their children need to do more than sit on a chair and drink Diet Coke—and they definitely shouldn't behave like General Patton.

Take the grandchildren out for a couple of hours to the mall or the movies. Bring dinner. Engage the grandchildren in a game of Chutes and Ladders. Your own children will be so happy to get their kids out of their hair for a brief time that they'll long for your next visit. And the beauty of children at this stage of life is that they are returnable. You get to leave anytime you want!

Move closer. Of course, to visit often it's easier if you live nearby, and in today's mobile society that's no easy thing. You might want to give some serious thought to repotting yourself to be closer to your family. William and Lillian Luby were determined to be mainstays in the lives of their two grandchildren, so they followed their daughter and her husband, Mary and Tim Fosnow, to three separate homes, buying a house and moving in up the block. The Fosnows couldn't have been more pleased because they had their own space, but the grandparents were always ready to babysit or otherwise help with the kids, who today have a wonderful relationship with their grandparents.

The Lubys are not all that unusual. Builders report a growing number of orders for two houses in the same development, one for the parents and one for the grandparents. Dr. Mohammed Jafferi, a retired physician in the Chicago area, bought an entire cul-de-sac where he and his four grown children moved into five separate single-family houses. While that is extreme, a Century21.com poll found that 51 percent responded "family" when asked whom they preferred as neighbors. Only 16 percent chose movie stars, and 12 percent chose athletes. Rock stars came in at the bottom of the list, at 6 percent.

Dealing with distance. For many there will be no escaping the fact that your children and grandchildren live far away. Frequent visits and great vacations will not be easy. That doesn't mean you have to give up on the relationship. Establish a set time each week to call your grandchildren. Make sure you speak to each one on each call, or alternate one per call for more meaningful conversations. Young children can be tough to get speaking, and they might clam up fast if all you have to say to them is that your back aches or ask how much they've grown. They'd rather talk about the dance recital or play they were just in, or about the home run they hit in Little League on Saturday.

They'll also listen and take an interest in you if you experience some of the same things they do. So make a point of seeing some of the same movies and watching a few of the same TV shows. Visit their favorite store. Read a book they are studying in school. Make good use of a fax machine or scanner to receive their artwork. Send postcards from every place you visit. E-mail often. If the children are young enough you might even record yourself reading bedtime stories and send them the tape. And when you do visit, make a point of spending a typical day with your grandchildren. See their favorite places and meet their friends. You'll find that you have plenty to talk about.

What Matters Most in Life?

Staying connected takes effort, whether it's with your kids and grandkids, a spouse, friend, or lover. But that effort is its own reward in that it keeps you active, engaged, and ageless while doing something nourishing for both your physical health and emotional well-being. You can't wait for the world to come to you.

Life has changed. Your kids are spread out and stressed out with their family and career foremost in their minds. Your friendships and maybe your marriage are being tested by your own longevity and ever evolving interests. Yet the old connections you value can be saved even as you begin new relationships. At this point in life, time is on your side. You have many healthy years ahead and the wisdom and opportunity to make the connections that are so vital to your happiness.

Ken had the pleasure of spending time with former president Carter a few years ago while assisting him in the development of his *Virtues of Aging* book. Ken reflects,

> I was dazzled by Carter's powerful and inquisitive mind, his kindness and extraordinary compassion. Seeking to glean some of his wisdom during one of our private visits, I asked President Carter what was the main difference in his view of the meaning of life now, in his seventies, versus twenty years ago. "When I was in my fifties," Carter told me, "I thought the things that mattered most were the things you could see—an expensive car, a big beautiful home, status, and wealth. Now I see that it's none of that. What truly matters in life are the things that you cannot see; the deep love you share with your family and close friends, your spiritual faith, the contributions you make to other people's lives, and your wealth of lifetime experiences are what really matter."

Those words strike us as a kind of existential North Star, and since we're all going to be charting new courses in the years ahead, a North Star or two can be very helpful. For decades we have lived our lives in a busy, competitive, and highly materialistic fashion. Don't get us wrong—we have great respect for productivity and the rewards and pleasure that money can buy—but as we're coming out of the vortex of our immature years, our center of gravity will migrate to our most valuable relationships and experiences. That's where the real gold is buried.

4

Creating Your New Dream Job

Some years ago Ken was asked to join a hundred Seattle retirees on a television show to discuss what the producer was calling the "new retirement." The show was to last sixty minutes, half of it an interview on the rapidly improving health and longevity of older adults, and half of it questions from the audience of retirees. As Ken tells the story:

> This is the kind of thing I enjoy doing. So I agreed, and when I arrived the producers excitedly told me there had been a lot of buzz building around the program. They were expecting good ratings. At that point, the studio doors burst open and to my surprise I saw not the legion of retirees I had been told would be attending but classroom upon classroom of six-year-olds flying to their seats, eager for a shot at being on TV. I wondered if I was in the wrong place.
>
> "Oh, my God," the executive producer yelled. "We've gotten our schedules reversed! The first-graders were

supposed to be here tomorrow for a show about amusement parks."

"Well, what should we do?" I asked.

"This is live TV," the producer returned. "We'll just have to talk with these kids about retirement. Let's do it!"

The show began with the cohosts asking me a wide range of questions about longevity and aging trends, and it generally went well. But the whole time my mind kept wandering to what would happen in the next segment when the kids started asking the questions. Would there even be any questions? But when that time finally came, lots of hands shot into the air, and the first question cut right to the heart of the matter. A little girl wanted to known how long she'd live. I think I delighted the kids by saying many of them would live to be a hundred. "Yay!" they all cheered.

But then a little boy somberly asked if he would be like his grandpa, who was sickly and unable to have much of a relationship with him. I tried to console the boy, saying that because of the miracles of modern medicine when it was his turn to be a grandpa he would look and feel a lot younger.

Then a little girl asked what job she would have when she was grown up. "Many," I said. "We may have three to seven careers through our life." "Yay!" The kids cheered again, really liking this idea. Picking up on their excitement, I said that in the future if people got stuck in one job and didn't like it anymore they would take a little time off and go back to school to learn something new. Then they'd start a whole new career. Hearing this, the kids started cheering louder than ever.

And that's the way the show on the new retirement model ended: with a rousing chorus of approval. The kids embraced their later years as an opportunity to do and be many things, and so do we.

Your power years are pregnant with possibilities, none more sweeping than new options for a more satisfying and less pressured balance of work and life. Certainly not all of us will want to work even part-time in our later years. But we won't view them as a permanent vacation either. We'll see this time as a turning point when we can take a break, take stock of who we are, and reinvent ourselves for the next chapter of life.

To make the most of this potential metamorphosis, it can be very helpful to start preparing today. Just as we began planning for our first career while we were in high school or college, we can spend time now—during our primary career years—building a foundation for whatever comes next, whether it's work for pay, volunteerism, a focus on family, or some long-obscured passion such as sculpting or working with animals.

If you're forty or fifty or even sixty, this chapter will help you identify and, when the time comes, land a satisfying power years career. Now is the time to reflect on what you've accomplished and build on it. Work that you enjoy is a proven source of psychological and physical well-being. The idea that you should give it up solely because you've reached a certain age is hopelessly retro. Even if your primary career has been unsatisfying, there's a good chance that in your power years you can find a job you love.

After thirty-seven years as a marketing executive at PG&E, Frank Dillon of Concord, California, retired with a generous pension and personal assets of more than $1 million. He spent his first golden year doing exactly as he had long envisioned—reading, playing some golf, and one by one, knocking off odd jobs and home improvements, including building a deck at his home. But then something he had not envisioned intruded on his years of preparation: he grew very bored. So he took a part-time job supervising tee times at a nearby golf club. "I just wanted something to do," Dillon explains. "I like to meet people and keep active." He eventually went back to work full-time as a consultant to his old employer for fulfillment, not out of need.

In this decision, Dillon has lots of company. Research shows that our generation heartily embraces the concept of extending our productive years. In the Merrill Lynch New Retirement Survey of more than three thousand boomers, only 17 percent said they intended to stop working for pay forever. Those who most wanted to stop working permanently tended to be men and women with less education and who had been working at low-paying or dull jobs. The first choice for the ideal work/leisure arrangement—picked by 42 percent of the generation—would be to be able to cycle in and out of work and leisure for extended periods throughout their lives. A smaller group, 16 percent, hoped to continue working part-time; 13 percent were planning on starting their own business; and 6 percent fully intend to keep working full-time right through their retirement years. One of the most fascinating insights from this study came from the fact that an incredible 56 percent of our generation who intend to keep working are hoping to do so in a completely new career or line of work!

Lest you think that this is just an American fad, in the recent HSBC-sponsored international study The Future of Retirement in a World of Rising Life Expectancies, for which eleven thousand people from all over the world were asked how they felt about working in retirement, there was total rejection of the idea of mandatory retirement (which is still legal in most countries). There was overwhelming agreement that maturity was not the beginning of the end and that old age had less to do with chronology than level of health and vitality. In addition, while people in places such as Brazil, Mexico, India, and Hong Kong were inclined to view life after retirement as primarily a time for rest and relaxation, in the United States, Canada, the United Kingdom, France, and China, respondents viewed these years as an "opportunity for a whole new chapter" in life. And perhaps in reflection of a true global trend, cycling between work and leisure emerged as the preferred new model for later life engagement in the majority of the areas surveyed (www .HSBC.com/futureofresearch).

Further, when asked why so many wanted to stay involved with work, in every study the overwhelming response was not the money. Instead, two in three say the main reason they want to keep working is to stay mentally active—twice the number of votes given to the economic motivations. Members of our highly educated and productive generation simply don't want to live a life of intellectual stagnation and mental irrelevance. According to Sir John Bond, Group Chairman of HSBC Holdings: "In this landmark study we have found that the people of the world are already creating their own solutions. For example, we found that people are not simply expecting to work longer, now they want to mix work and leisure, learning and rest. And it is critical that governments, regulators, corporations and financial institutions understand these emerging trends in behavior and attitude if we are to successfully tackle the pressing issues before us."

Work is clearly an important part of our continuing plans. But work in our power years will be very different and can be far more rewarding.

It also may be difficult to decide just what you want to do. Russell Rosenberg, fifty, finds himself at a bittersweet turning point. He's put in a successful twenty-five years in the clothing industry, the last eleven as one of two partners importing apparel from Asia and reselling to some of the biggest retail chains. In all those years, though, Rosenberg never really enjoyed his work even though it provided him with the resources to live well, raise two sons and support his wife, save for retirement, and, upon selling out to his partner recently, secure enough income to support his lifestyle for at least five years.

"The real story here is I got into a business I did not have a passion for," he says. "When I was young I went to school as a film and photography major and drove a taxi part-time for five years while working as a photo studio assistant. I longed for a career with greater financial stability. Soon enough my girlfriend who was a textile designer and friends of mine in the clothing business urged me to get a steady gig. So I kind of got into that business in spite of myself."

He has every intention of returning to work. His boys are still at home and within a few years he'll need the income. But he doesn't want to back into another occupation. "I resisted the urge to quit all those years when I was traveling six months a year and doing something I had no passion for. Now I'm finally free from that brain-dead feeling. I badly wanted this opportunity to not spend the rest of my life going through the motions."

He is just beginning to search for his hidden passions, and he confides that the search is not an easy one. He signed up for a film course, but quickly found that he had outgrown his onetime interest in making movies. He ordered books and tapes on how to trade stocks, and while those have helped him manage his money better, they have not sparked an interest in full-time trading. He's also begun visiting galleries, attending art auctions, and collecting photographs. There he's at least found a spark. He loves photography; opening a small gallery would let him enjoy that pastime while playing to his entrepreneurial strengths. "At this point I know I can't go to work for someone else," he says. "And I can't stay at home, where I just get distracted by domestic tasks. Since I was a kid I was always very industrious. At college I started a trucking business, moving student luggage. I was always entrepreneurial. Ultimately I believe that will wind up happening again. I'll do something that will utilize my business background."

But getting focused has not been easy. Even the photo gallery idea leaves him less than fully inspired. "Everybody says to me you should be pursuing your passion," Rosenberg says. "But nothing is really presenting itself. This is a toughie."

Reach Your Potential

In your primary career you've probably been focused on one version or another of climbing the corporate ladder. You've been burdened with the costs of setting up a household, raising children, putting them through college, paying down the mortgage, and paying off your credit cards. Maybe you've needed to squeeze out every dime of pay, even if it's meant working at something you haven't enjoyed, just to make ends meet. Lost in this dog-eat-dog existence may have been any sense of what your true calling may be. That notion has been suppressed as you focused on the needs of your family and getting ahead at the office.

If you liberate yourself from the belief that work in your powers years must mean staying at what you do longer than you'd like, the picture gets far more interesting. A banker can become a teacher; a *Fortune* 500 executive can turn a hobby into a small business; an accountant can become a bartender; a doctor can become a motivational speaker. If you've saved enough, maybe you'll devote time to running a volunteer ambulance service.

In your maturity, you can count on:

Heightened self-awareness. We're not kids anymore; we've lived and we've learned. We can look back on many years of experiences that have given us insights into who we are, what we do well, and what we love to do. By now we have learned that happiness doesn't come from doing what others think we should do but from following our heart to what we most enjoy.

Expanded capacity for risk. As we enter this new stage of life we will leave behind many of the fears and obligations that formerly constrained us. Most of us will no longer have to prove ourselves on the job as we did when we were younger. We've built a storehouse of confidence and goodwill and can try new things without worrying about ridicule or reprisal should we stumble. This is the perfect time to shed our limitations and become the person we always wanted to be. Joan Schweighardt did it. In her late fifties she founded GreyCore Press, a publishing company. "I doubt I would have done it had I been younger," she says. "There is a certain sense of freedom that aging brings and a lack of concern about the possibility of failure."

Diminishing financial responsibilities. Our children likely will have left home, and most other expenses related to rearing and educating them will be behind us. Many other expenses, such as the monthly mortgage payment, also may have disappeared. Assuming we've saved something along the way, we should be able to easily manage our power years on one-half to two-thirds of what we made in our primary career years.

Lifestyle flexibility. With fewer responsibilities you will have more freedom to work the hours of the day and days of the week you prefer and to relocate wherever you want to pursue your dreams. You'll have the opportunity to build your career around core passions and your most compelling talents. Instead of retiring and stopping work altogether, you can choose the projects that excite you. Jerry Fournier, fifty-five, of Farmington Hills, Michigan, is an executive vice president of HDS Services, a food-service company. His children are grown and he has saved enough to quit work anytime he likes. But he's not even thinking about it. He enjoys work too much and points out that his lifestyle model is his company's chairman, who comes to work chipper every day at age eighty-eight.

Why Work?

Behavioral psychologist Abraham Maslow asserted five fundamental human needs: survival, security, belonging, self-esteem, and self-actualization. Think about those needs for just a moment and you realize that work can have a role in satisfying every single one. Maslow argued that these basic human needs are hierarchical, meaning that you must satisfy each one before moving up the chain to a higher need. Briefly, let's look at Maslow's progression.

The first level is survival: food, shelter and clothing. Our jobs certainly give us the means to meet those needs. The second level is security. Work gives us that in two ways: it provides the financial resources we need to secure our lifestyle, and it also makes us feel like we belong somewhere, the third level, lending our lives the stability and predictability that we feel we need. There is a sense of security that comes with waking up in the morning and knowing that we have a purpose and a place to be, and what to expect when we get there. Most of us say the workplace provides our primary connection with friends and society; one in three say we meet most of our friends at the office. Workplace connections are what drive Bob Harrell of Seymour, Indiana, to stay on the job. Harrell, ninety-two, works twelve-hour days as a highway and bridge engineer. "I'm trying to cut back," he says. "But I have so many friends at work, and I can't really leave them." Sixty-five percent of today's working elders say they stay at work mainly to keep up with friendships. Many consider the chance to stay in touch with young coworkers a bonus.

The fourth level is self-esteem. According to Maslow, when we excel and achieve we experience feelings of self-confidence, worth, strength, capability, and adequacy; of being useful and necessary in the world. On the other hand, when we fail or even fail to try, we experience feelings of inferiority, weakness, and helplessness. Work is our primary proving ground. In adulthood work gives us our best chance to flex our mental muscles and be recognized for what we do well. People who do well at their jobs and then quit are prone to diminishing self-esteem in later life. So if for no other reason we should rethink any ideas we may have of retiring early or entirely.

Brian Naber was the president of a small steel company in Burlington, Ontario, before he retired at age fifty-five. "My idea was to turn all my efforts to my hobbies," he says. "I do wood-carving, woodworking, and landscaping. I have lots of interests to keep me busy." But less than a year into retirement, Naber changed his mind. "As time was going on, I was getting more bored and less self-fulfilled," he says. A life of leisure simply did not work for him, and within a few years he had launched his own small business in Cincinnati, Ohio.

The capstone of Maslow's hierarchy is self-actualization. As he explained, "Even if all other needs are satisfied a new discontent and restlessness [may] develop, unless the individual is doing what he or she, individually, is fitted for. Musicians must make music, artists must paint, poets must write, if they are to be ultimately at peace with themselves. What humans can be, they must be."

Being self-actualized means doing what we are truly cut out to do. It's an honest convergence of work and play in which our work is no longer labor but an enjoyment, the highest expression of who and what we desire to be. Few get there. But because we'll live so long we have a unique opportunity to seek and find Maslow's version of nirvana.

You may have missed your true calling early in life or been under too much pressure to explore the possibilities. Your power years can be your chance to create a career that allows you to fulfill your core passions. Work can shift from something you must do to something you love to do. Ophthalmologist Herve M. Bryon launched a new career as a medical expert on

TV after he retired from medicine. "I have seen many individuals retire at various ages," he says. "Those who anticipate little more than playing golf, fishing, traveling, or just hanging around with their other retired friends invariably become unhappy, bored, and cynical. On the other hand, I have observed people who carefully planned a transition into a completely new field or a different area of expertise within their profession or business. Inevitably, they became dynamic, productive, and desirable in their new status. What could be more gratifying than to apply all the wisdom that comes with increasing years to a new challenge?"

Dan recalls the early retirement dreams of one of his boyhood friends, Dave, who Dan checked in with recently after having lost touch years ago:

Dave, who like me is approaching fifty, seared his way into my brain more than thirty years ago with an audacious pledge to retire early. We were probably twenty at the time, not yet finished with college at different universities. Neither of us had ever held a job much longer than spring break, and yet one summer night after tipping a third or fourth beer Dave confidently aired his early-retirement aspirations: "I want to knock myself out, make as much money as I can, and retire at forty-five. Life is too short. I don't want to spend my time slaving away for someone else."

If anyone could retire at forty-five—without an inheritance or unearned windfall—I figured it was Dave. He was always the most popular kid in class; he starred as the high school quarterback and did it effortlessly. He seemed to have guardian angels perpetually looking over both shoulders. Other than an afternoon of golf at a high school reunion some years ago, I hadn't seen or spoken to Dave in two decades, but I thought of him and his outrageous pledge shortly after starting work on this book. Mostly, I was flat curious if he'd done it. But I also wondered if, like many of us, he had found financial freedom difficult to achieve, or if just possibly he had changed his worldview.

So I called him at his home in St. Louis and asked. It turns out Dave's track was a little slower than his earlier vision. "But I almost made it," he told me. "I've been in the trucking business all my life and when I was thirty-seven years old, with fifteen years under my belt, I took my shot just like I always figured. I went to work on straight commission for a guy who ran a transportation consulting firm. I was on track to earn $600,000 my fourth year, which would have gotten me pretty close. But the guy realized there was nothing in my contract to keep him from letting me go and hiring someone cheap to manage the accounts I'd brought in, and that's just what he did." Dave is back on salary for another freight firm. "I've still got two kids to put through college, so now I'm shooting for fifty-eight or sixty."

But Dave's worldview has changed, too. As he ponders his power years, he still dreams of a second home on a lake with a bass boat, and of traveling through Europe with his wife, Mary, whom he started dating in seventh grade. Yet work is no longer a time thief that he wants desperately to put behind bars so he can get on with what he really enjoys. Work has become part of what gives him satisfaction each day. "If I can stay involved in what I'm doing now on a consulting basis without pressure and at my leisure, that's what I'll do. You can make a lot of money if you get set up right, and this work is something I really enjoy. It's still a thrill for me to close a big sale."

The Coming Power Years Job Boom

What kind of jobs will be out there for us? Will employers ease up on their preference for young blood? Will workforce ageism diminish? We wouldn't preach the merits of staying at work longer if your options were limited to bagging groceries or grilling burgers on the night shift. However, this is a circumstance where demography is destiny, because a glance into the population tea leaves reveals that over the next ten years a severe shortage of seasoned workers will develop as members of our generation begin to leave the workforce. The baby bust generation behind us is just too small to fill all the jobs we will be vacating, and Generation X will be lacking in the kind of experience, knowledge, and management firepower we have accumulated over the years. In all sorts of careers, from nursing to nuclear engineering, there simply aren't enough skilled people in the pipeline to fill the coming void. For these reasons, increasing numbers of companies will entice us to stay on longer through a grab bag of benefits, concessions, and special scheduling that will seem too good to be true.

Remember that the number of North American workers under age forty-five exploded by forty million in the '70s and '80s, as we boomers entered the workforce. Not surprisingly, the hiring strategies and benefits policies of employers back then were geared toward the young and centered on things such as advancement potential and, for women, decent maternity leaves. As we got ahead in our companies, the focus shifted to policies that made it easier for us to secure our financial future through 401(k) plans and portable pensions. By the 1990s, the influx of boomers had run its course. The youngest were over thirty; we were all already at work. Late in the decade, for the first time, companies began to contemplate their future due to a shrinking pool of young workers. Charles Romeo, the head of human resources at the giant food processor ConAgra, noted that "this is not a temporary situation. It is a fact of life. Some companies may be in denial, but we are way past that."

IBM, Monsanto, Borders Books, GE, Starbucks, Deloitte Consulting, CVS pharmacies, Days Inn, Citigroup, Home Depot, and Xerox are leaders in creating flexible job schedules for workers over age fifty-five. These and other forward thinking companies are being rewarded with a surprisingly enthusiastic pool of mature workers that is far larger than they initially figured. At an Older Worker Job Fair in Orange County, California, event organizers had prepared for a crowd of no more than a hundred. When some five hundred mature job seekers arrived, the twenty-three employers hosting the event quickly ran out of applications.

This talent pool will continue to expand. Employers will increasingly fight to keep talented older workers. They'll do this with an array of benefits such as better health coverage and portable financial accounts that appeal to the new breed of employee who wants to cycle in and out of work. The 401(k) plans were designed for our savings years and don't hold great appeal for those who are already at an age when they are taking distributions. Among the new wrinkles we expect will be the elimination of government and employer disincentives to continue working on the one hand and more financial offerings that allow us to keep our money in tax-favored plans longer, without mandatory withdrawals, and new accounts that allow us to cycle in and out of our savings plans in conjunction with our work schedules. We'll be able to take withdrawals when we're not working and make contributions again when we are working.

Flexible work schedules and flex-retirement will continue to become common—not just for the busy, caregiving mom, but also for the can't-wait-to-go-fishing older worker. Currently, some 40 percent of U.S. employers allow staff to work from home, up from 20 percent five years ago; 75 percent offer flexible hours, a 17 percent increase over ten years ago. Two in five companies now have job sharing arrangements, where two or more part-timers fill a single full-time slot. "What we don't want to see happen is people leaving the company because they just can't make their schedules work," says Debra Capolarello, senior vice president of human resources for MetLife. "That's not the position that we want to be in. We want to be proactive about using alternative work arrangements as a tool to attract and retain our talent."

Can older workers get the job done? Thankfully, yes. Not only are we staying healthy longer, but also, as the industrial age has given way to the information age, our economy has transformed from one based on physical production to one based on knowledge and service. By 2025 the U.S. government projects that service will account for 85 percent of jobs. Every day that work becomes less physically demanding it becomes better suited to seasoned adults with years of stored knowledge. There is also good news in the fact that much of the bias toward hiring and retaining younger workers—and avoiding older ones—is based on myth. In the New Employer/Employee Equation Survey of seventy-five hundred U.S. workers that Age Wave conducted in collaboration with the Concours Group, older workers turned out to be the most satisfied, the most engaged in their work, and the least likely to feel burned out. In stark contrast, younger workers were the most distressed and restless and felt the least amount of loyalty to their employers. In addition, since more mature workers are also more loyal and committed, an employer's investment in a committed fifty-year-old is likely to get a better return on investment than in a twenty-one-year-old, who's far more likely to hop jobs repeatedly. It also turns out that younger workers are more likely to feel dead-ended in their careers than older ones.

In the spring of 2001, *Fortune* magazine analyzed a wide

sample of stock pickers, analysts, and brokers, and correlated the results by years in the financial industry. Going in, there was an assumption that young "new economy" analysts would be the most tuned in to new economy market trends. But the opposite was true. During the twelve-month period from March 2000 through February 2001, amid the worst bear market in decades as the S&P 500 fell 21.6 percent the stock picks of analysts who had been on the job less than four years lost a worse-than-average 23 percent, which was far worse than the 13 percent lost by analysts on the job between four and ten years. That, in turn, was far worse than the 8 percent lost by analysts on the job ten to twenty years. Those on the job more than twenty years did best: they lost just 5.5 percent. As we age, employers will seek boomers who have kept up our skills regardless of when we were born. "Employability has a lot to do with our mind," asserts Donald P. Kennedy, chairman of First American Financial Corp. He should know. He is eighty-three.

Discover Your Next Calling

Imagine waking up every morning looking forward to doing whatever you most enjoy. This may not be easy. Caught up in your current career and family for so many years, you may not remember where your true passions lie. It's time to rediscover them, and some new ones as well.

Start by writing down every job you've had since you first cut the lawn or shoveled snow. Under each job list three things about the job that you most enjoyed. These would be the things you most looked forward to each morning and reflected on each night. When you were doing these things, time flew by and you may have worked late or on the weekends to complete them. They may even have been the only things that kept you in a job you otherwise disliked.

In Dan's case, he's always suffered the meetings and various other planning functions necessary in the editorial world, hopefully (but not always) with a smile. But the simple act of putting words on paper has been his absolute joy. He's been a journalist for twenty-five years. On his list would be: writing, speaking with interesting people, spotting important trends, and communicating to others information that can help them (and cowriting this book). At this writing Dan is forty-nine and is just beginning to think about his power years. The things he enjoys about journalism could lead him down many roads, including writing fiction, opening a pub to interact with different kinds of people, or coaching a basketball team to satisfy his urge to impart knowledge. He thinks he might even be able to do all three!

In Ken's case, the things he loves most are learning new things, creating new ideas and solutions, and sharing them with others. What he likes least are the bureaucratic meetings (you can see how the authors found each other!), tedious or repetitive work, and working with uninspired clients. As a result, when he reinvented his career at age fifty (five years ago), he shed all the layers of responsibility and tedium that wore him down and turned his attentions to conducting breakthrough research, seeking out exciting new clients and business partners, stepping up his public speaking involvements, and cowriting this book. In addition, recognizing his need for more quality time with his family, he opted to work less and take more time off for fun and play.

When making your list, don't rule out anything. You may be surprised at how much you've done in your life and what parts of your jobs have given you the most satisfaction. Maybe it was managing employees or serving as a mentor to young workers, or talking to customers, planning or hosting company parties, carpooling, writing memos, organizing files, surfing the Internet, or just chatting at the water cooler. All of these hold clues to your core passions. You may notice one or two things that appear over and over in various forms. That's good. It can help you quickly focus on what you really like to do.

All the Things You Like to Do

Now repeat the exercise for any volunteer work you've been involved with, and then for how you've spent your leisure hours. Think about what motivated your interests to begin with and what parts you've most enjoyed. Look also at your spiritual and social lives and your friendships. Sometimes how you pray and play tells as much about your true self as how you work. What kind of people have you most enjoyed spending time with? What kinds of contacts have been most satisfying? What activities and events have you most enjoyed?

Even though this may sound odd, make a list of how you spend discretionary income. The way you choose to use your limited resources is a good indicator of your priorities. Where do you most like to shop? Do your spending patterns reveal that you love entertainment, sports, beauty supplies, electronics, do-it-yourself projects? Do they show a person who loves people-oriented pastimes or quiet, reflective pleasures?

Your choices through the first fifty years of life can inform and inspire your blueprint for what comes next. For twenty years Tim Tingle ran New Canaan Farms, a gourmet food manufacturer in Dallas, Texas, where he was known for end-lessly telling interesting stories to motivate his employees. "At every company gathering, I would tell hero stories of employ-ees who had gone far beyond what was expected and achieved success," Tingle recalls. "These stories were my first awakening to the power of stories to motivate and bring out the hero in us all." In 1990, the Texas Department of Agriculture asked Tingle to put on a series of workshops for small agricultural companies. As he prepared for these talks, Tingle reflected on his techniques and came to the transformative realization that storytelling, not business management, was what most fasci-nated him.

"This was the true beginning of my second career, as a story-teller," Tingle says. These days he's having the time of his life each year telling stories onstage at hundreds of schools, festivals, and universities throughout the country. Under the sponsorship of the Department of Defense, he has toured Germany five times and was recently the keynote speaker at the Heidelberg Young Authors Conference. His collection of Native American stories for kindergarten through fifth grade, *Grandma Spider Brings the Fire*, was nominated for a Storytelling World Award. His most popular work, *The Choctaw Way*, features traditional and historical stories and chants of this Native American culture. As Tingle reflects, "I sold New Canaan Farms in 1997 and have never been happier in my life. I am doing what I was put on earth to do."

Remembering the Dreams of Your Youth

Now it's time for another list. Take a minute to think back to your childhood. And, if you can, hunt through some of your old report cards, letters to and from friends, or diary entries. What did you dream about doing with your life? Write down every-thing you remember about those dreams and ask yourself how you may have kept them alive in your work, hobbies, or recre-ation. Although your joys may have evolved, many people find this exercise to be a powerful starting point for recovering their core passions. Remembering the first things you wanted to do with your life can provide invaluable insight, especially if you feel that your dreams have been obscured by the struggle to sur-vive and raise a family over the past thirty years. Dan was going through the attic recently and chanced upon his eighth-grade graduation program. He had long forgotten that he originally wanted to be a TV sports commentator. In his case, he never strayed far from his core passion of communicating information and opinion. Knowing your personal North Star can help guide you to your own next chapter.

Most people stray, so don't be discouraged if you find that you have, too. When she was growing up, Helena Hale had a passion for acting. She majored in drama in college and landed several roles on Broadway. But she gave it all up after having children so that she could earn a steady living as a schoolteacher. After many years as an educator, and as she was contemplating retirement, Hale recalled her passion for the stage and began taking parts in community theater. Now retired, she travels the country as an actress and is more inspired than she was 50 years ago. "I become more and more of an artist the longer I do this," she says.

Your Greatest Hits

Review your career one more time, this time looking for moments of greatness—when you knew you had hit your stride and felt as if you were, as they say in sports, in the zone. This might have been a time when you were widely recognized by peers or when you just enjoyed what you were doing in relative anonymity. Identify what made these times so wonderful. If you were part of a team, what role did you play? Were you the captain, or did you prefer to be the scorekeeper? What skills and personality traits came alive during these endeavors? Did you take risks, did you venture into something new, did you master a skill that had previously intimidated you, or did you demonstrate courage or persistence? Did you experience these greatest moments alone or did your satisfaction arise out of being involved with a group? What kind of a group was it? How did you relate to the members? What did you enjoy about being with them?

Think of these peak moments as the highlights or greatest hits of your life. Identifying them can provide clues to your true ambitions and can help you position yourself to become exactly who you want to be. In a later step you'll assemble a wide-ranging team of helpers to move you along through their contacts and insights. But initially you should reach out to family and friends who have insights into the things you do best and love most. Be honest. Explain to your loved ones that you are trying to rediscover your core passions and fashion a new career or later-life pursuit that will keep you fulfilled. Ask them to share the moments when they believed you were most excited or happy. Then sit back and listen.

You may be surprised by what you hear—and later by what you accomplish. Don Davidson of Wilton, Connecticut, converted his lifelong hobby into a custom woodworking business after a thirty-year career in publishing—after consulting with his children and grandchildren, who got so excited about his new venture that they became his business partners. If he ever does retire, he expects that his grandsons will take over.

Take Advantage of Community Resources

Career coaches and placement firms provide excellent insight and guidance. Most community colleges offer vocational testing. Many have evaluation systems that can help you discover the kind of environment where you function best. You can also take an interest-assessment test, such as the Strong-Campbell Interest Inventory or the Kuder Occupational Interest Survey. Vocational aptitude tests, including the Differential Aptitude Test and the General Aptitude Test Battery, can give you insight into your evolving late-life ambitions.

George Rogers, retired after thirty years as a straight-arrow engineer for the U.S. Navy, took stock of himself at age fifty-eight and concluded that he wasn't ready to drop out of circulation. But he was confused about what came next until he finished a vocational aptitude exam at a nearby community college. To his surprise, he found that he scored well in applied arts and commercial design, things that had interested him in his teens but that he had forgotten. Now he is a commercial artist telecommuting twenty to forty hours a week from his home in Asheville, North Carolina. "I feel like I've died and gone to heaven," he says. "I can't get enough."

Eckerd College in St. Petersburg, Florida, always an innovator in educational programs for adults, offers a Program for Experienced Learners, where students receive college credit for skills acquired in the workplace and can take classes on a flexible schedule. Westchester Community College in Valhalla, New York, has a program called Mainstream, which helps older adults identify career options.

Your Vision Statement

Envisioning what you want is the critical first step toward making your dreams come true. Key to unlocking this vision is making the effort to think things through and then putting down on paper what you discover about yourself. The value of writing down your observations should not be underestimated. Putting your thoughts on paper forces you to distill them into clear statements and goals. It also helps your loved ones and other helpers understand you and get a better feel for what you're trying to do. So as part of this exercise, when you've reached some conclusions about exactly what makes you happy and fulfilled, write down a vision statement. The statement should be one paragraph that summarizes what you are good at, where your core passions lie, and how you plan to fuse the two in later life.

Here are some sample vision statements:

I am a terrific salesperson and I love selling people things that will make their lives better. Although in recent years I've been a manager, the truth is I haven't enjoyed it. I intend to find a small to midsize real estate or insurance company where I can have a blast by turning on all of my selling engines and making a good living in the process. However, because I also enjoy playing golf and fishing, I will only work three days each week!

I am an accomplished executive who gets great satisfaction from fixing problems and helping employees achieve great things. I like to manage a project and then move on quickly to the next challenge. It doesn't matter to me if it's with a *Fortune* 500 company, my church, or the Red Cross. I intend to find a series of organizations that will let me jump in as needed. And because I enjoy mentoring, I will be especially interested in working with younger people or volunteers who are open to being coached.

I am a caring and successful manager who is well organized and enjoys working with people from varied backgrounds. I get frustrated by bureaucratic organizations. So I intend to help entrepreneurs in my community develop and manage viable businesses. And because I am a woman who was brought up poor and have discovered that I am most appreciated by women who started with modest means, I will focus on highly motivated young women from the inner city.

Throughout my life I have worked in an office, but during my free time I have always enjoyed the outdoors. I am going to find a way to get a job—even for no pay—where I can spend all of my time outside, surrounded by nature. Maybe I will volunteer at the local campgrounds or state park.

Although I have been a bookkeeper my whole life, what I really like to do is take care of other people, especially older adults. I love seeing my efforts make others feel more comfortable and loved. So I will seek a job where I can help others as an elder care provider at a local senior center or assisted living facility.

Your vision statement should resonate with your core desires and fill you with excitement. If you pursue your honest-to-goodness passion you can create a new power years career that not only provides a helpful paycheck but also satisfies your need for personal growth.

Exploring Your New Career Options

Once you have defined your core passions and talents, you are ready to explore your strategies for bringing them to life. If your vision includes work, you have three basic options: (1) remain with your current employer but in a flexible role that fits your lifestyle and allows you to focus on the things that excite you; (2) go to a new employer to pursue your passions in a different setting; or (3) start your own business around the things you enjoy. Let's look at these one at a time.

1. Staying with Your Longtime Employer

You may not be sure if your boss likes you much, but if you're getting the job done, he or she probably will want you to stick around. As we've mentioned, companies are bending some of the rules and creating many new ones to accommodate the fifty-plus set these days, offering phased retirement, part-time work, job sharing, consulting, flexible hours, work from home, and project-based assignments. Even if your company hasn't yet gotten religion on the need to hire or retain older workers and has yet to institutionalize any of these new job arrangements, you may be able use the information in this section to talk your boss into getting with the trend. Among companies that are moving most aggressively to keep their older talent are Home Depot, Borders, Wal-Mart, Pitney-Bowes, MetLife, and Walgreens. Consultant William M. Mercer found that:

- 47 percent of companies allow older workers to reduce their hours

- 42 percent of companies hire older workers on a temporary basis

- 42 percent retain retiring workers as consultants

- 17 percent allow job sharing for older workers

Mercer found that 45 percent of companies have special positions for adults including job training and mentoring. More than half of the companies in the Mercer study said they were willing to negotiate special arrangements for older workers. For example, standard corporate policy prohibits the straight rehiring of recent company retirees. But some managers have gone so far as to refer a valued former employee to a temp agency, to be placed back in the company he or she retired from. Managers also increasingly bring back retirees as consultants or independent contractors. If this is the only way to stay with your company, don't take it personally. Innovation comes slowly.

You'll get your best deal by researching what other companies are doing and using this information to cut a deal with your employer, showing how it's in the firm's best interest to keep and motivate seasoned workers. Here are some examples of how leading-edge companies are managing this issue:

At Aerospace Corporation, without ever leaving the office, mature workers can downscale to part-time or self-employed consultants, or stick around full-time but take unpaid leaves of absence three months each year. They also can become a "retiree casual," which is the most popular option and allows them to retire with full pension and medical benefits and then be rehired for up to a thousand hours a year. "We have retiree casuals who are sixty-five, seventy-five, eighty years old and still working," says Charlotte Lazar-Morrison, the company's director of human resources. "They want to stay involved. It allows you to have people ready and available to work when we're in a surge mode. We can call them in and they can work when they feel like it." At any given time, about five hundred retiree casuals are signed up and about two hundred are at work, she says. Over the years, thousands of mature workers have participated in the program.

Cigna's Encore program allows older workers to log up to eighty hours a month and collect partial employment benefits as well as retiree benefits. Many of the nearly two hundred older adults who take advantage of this option each year work in the same departments they left.

At Monsanto, older workers are handed special projects to be completed on a flexible schedule. These workers are expected to pass on their technical knowledge to younger workers in the process. Employees may take up to six months off after "retiring" and then return to work up to a thousand hours a year. About six hundred former employees participate in the program. Some job-share. But most work two days a week. "We introduced phased retirement a decade ago because coming out of the lean and mean era of the 1980s we realized that we would need replacements and that we had qualified, intelligent, and loyal retirees whom we wanted to maintain our relationship with," says Liz Thien, head of the company's Retiree Resource Corps. Her staff of five includes four former retirees. "Since its inception in 1991, we have saved millions of dollars," Thien added. "And because the program is completely by choice, we get the best-motivated people."

At Deloitte Consulting, "senior partners" can customize their job, choosing how many hours they want to work, where they want to work, and which projects they want to work on.

Technology research company MITRE allows mature workers who have been with the company ten years to join its Reserves at the Ready program, through which they get a reduced schedule and work on projects that enable them to mentor young workers and pass along their knowledge of clients.

By the way, if your manager or human resources director is not familiar with these kinds of innovative approaches to retaining older workers, it's time they were. Lend them a copy of this book!

2. Finding a New Job with a New Employer

This isn't nearly as easy as staying put, but for many people it's a far more liberating move. You probably have not had a chance to prove yourself to outside employers, and you may be unfamiliar with the options you'll be exploring. But remember: with fewer obligations you're not so much trying to fit into a job; you can instead work to fit a job around who you really are or would like to become. Some things about your new career will seem strange, so establish priorities.

What do you value most? Flexible work almost certainly means hopping off the corporate ladder, possibly reporting to someone younger, and downshifting into a role with less prestige and lower pay. Get over it. Those are precisely the concerns you must shed to enjoy your power years career. It also provides opportunities to meet new people and learn new ideas, and you can even leave stuff behind if you're open to truly reinventing yourself. In surveys, very few older workers say they are primarily motivated by pay. What charges their batteries? Making a contribution, having fun, and being part of a team are far more rewarding than a big salary in a crummy job. Maybe you've already been there and done that.

Think creatively about how different businesses could use your skills, bearing in mind that you have a lot more to offer than can be captured on a one-page resumé. If, for example, you have been a schoolteacher and have a yen for communicating difficult subjects, you could become a health-care educator at a medical clinic or a financial planner at a bank. There may be limits to what you can do in your power years, but they are defined only by the extent to which you are willing to explore and learn new things. And learning is getting easier all the time. Community colleges usually have terrific computer, accounting, writing, and other training courses. Meanwhile, take advantage of the extra training available where you work now. Half of all large companies pay for courses that upgrade the skills of older workers.

3. Start Your Own Business

Becoming an entrepreneur is an increasingly popular choice. One in three mature adults who work currently does so at a small business they own. Free from many financial and most parental responsibilities and bolstered by the accumulated savings of a lifetime, many men and women finally take on the enjoyable risks of running their own shop. Why not? In your power years you bring to bear a battery of assets that are enormously valuable: contacts inside and outside your field, people skills honed over many years, practical experience, wisdom, and credibility. And, you don't really need to create an empire—free yourself from that kind of pressure. This is a time in life to enjoy what you do.

Starting a business can sometimes be challenging and risky. You won't have time to rebuild your assets if the venture fails, so you must make certain that you'll be able to handle the financial risks, and because starting a company is time-consuming, you must make sure this option is a good fit with the kind of lifestyle you seek. More than a few people have started a small business seeking a pleasant balance of work and leisure only to find the demands of running their company quickly consumed their life.

On the other hand, you might find yourself wildly successful as an entrepreneur. McDonald's origins date to 1955, when at the power years age of fifty-two Ray Kroc packed up the six-spindled milkshake mixers he was selling and visited California, where he was intrigued with the fast-food hamburger restaurant operated by Dick and Mac McDonald. Believing that there was a revolution in food service on its way and although many people thought he was crazy, Kroc purchased the rights to the name McDonald's and opened his first store in Des Plaines, Illinois, that year. From that modest beginning, McDonald's has become the largest fast-food business in the world, serving people at thirty-one thousand restaurants in 118 countries and with annual revenues in excess of $17 billion. Kroc never finished high school and didn't become successful until he was past sixty years old.

If starting your own company is your destiny, start laying the foundation now. It's never too soon to start. Ed was a high school teacher for thirty-four years. Toward the end of that career, he decided he wanted to open his own massage therapy spa. By learning the skills and beginning his business incrementally, while still teaching, he was able to build sustainable revenue by the time he quit teaching for good. "I started my postretirement business some ten years before I stopped teaching," he notes. "My advice to anyone over forty is plan ahead. These years come real quick."

Don't be shy about asking for help. To maximize the likelihood of success, you'll want to draw on all resources at your disposal, including family, friends, and business contacts. In addition, there are many organizations that help business start-ups. Anne Kleine, a career nurse, found invaluable help at the Service Corps of Retired Executives (SCORE) (www.score.org), a nonprofit organization comprised of retired executives who advise small-business owners. After hanging up her white shoes she sought help in setting up a small food company, and at SCORE she found two counselors who had experience in food distribution, patenting, and trademarks. With the help and encouragement of her team she created a business plan for Mrs. Kleine's Krelish, a condiment based on an old family recipe for sweet sauerkraut with onions, red bell peppers, spices, and sugar. Anne negotiated with a producer in Portland, Oregon, to plan an ambitious production and rollout. Her condiments are now at specialty stores throughout the Northwest. Anne's advice: "Keep your ears open. Listen to your mentors and advisers and always listen to your heart, not your head."

Make It Reality

Now it's time to turn your vision into reality. Put together a team of contacts to motivate and advise you. Don't try to go it alone. Having a team is much more effective and fun. You probably have a broad base of relatives, friends, and colleagues. Lean on them to introduce you to their friends and contacts, and keep building a network. You might even look up old friends and colleagues with whom you've lost touch. That's the advantage of thinking about your power years career now: you have time to develop key relationships with professional associates, customers, suppliers, and business partners who could be helpful later. Today's client could be tomorrow's investor. Today's vendor could be tomorrow's partner. Today's boss could be tomorrow's employee.

Because money planning is so important in launching a business, you may want a financial adviser on your team. You may also find that a personal coach or career counselor could be helpful. The other people you recruit for your team will depend on the nature of your goals. If you're going back to school and plan to change careers, include people who know about education and others in your new field. In the end, though, your spouse, kids, relatives, and close friends typically form the core of any effective support team. These are the people who know you best and care most about your welfare. Don't overlook their ability to contribute as you sort out your new ambitions.

To put together an advice team, start with all the people you count on for support right now. Your list might include your spouse, clergyman, best friend, favorite uncle, financial planner, lawyer, or maybe your ex-boss. Contact each of them and explain what you are trying to do and how you hope they can help. Use your vision statement to share what you have discovered about yourself and what you want to do with the rest of your life. Next go through your Rolodex looking for colleagues, customers, and other professional acquaintances who might be helpful and do the same with them. That might be a little tougher. If you don't get the response you want, try the next person on the list and focus your networking efforts on getting the kind of help you want.

Once your support team is in place—or even better, while you're still assembling it—put together a plan and a timetable for getting into the new career you choose. If planning isn't your strength, get help from someone on the support team who's good at it. A plan is critical, as Jonathan Saunders, a San Francisco advertising executive, learned. Saunders spent most of his life working hard and earning steady promotions. But he never gave a thought to mapping out the career he truly wanted. "My career was something that just kind of happened to me," he says. In his fifties, he realized that he didn't want to retire but he also knew that he wanted to try something different. "In my free time, I raced sailboats on the bay," he says. "As a skipper, you are constantly making decisions about the best course to follow, adjusting to the wind, currents, and tactics of the other boats. The best skipper is the one who thinks ahead and plans out the best course. Although I had never applied this strategy to my career, I realized that's what I needed to do to chart a new course for my life."

After much soul searching and discussions with close friends, Saunders realized his dream job would be one that married his two passions—boating and sales—so he decided to explore opening a boat store. "It was a little daunting," he says. "I didn't have any experience in retail." He started talking with other boating enthusiasts, retailers, and friends. "Like charting a sailing course, I developed a three-year plan to get into the industry. I started when I was fifty-eight and by the time I was sixty-one I was the proud proprietor of a small boating supply store. It took a lot of discipline and hard work but the careful planning and preparation took most of the anxiety out of the process. Now, instead of retiring and moping around the house all day, I've created a whole new job and a whole new life for myself."

Everyone's needs are different. But your plan doesn't need to be complicated. Start by determining how much time you have. If you're in your forties, you could have twenty years to prepare and can be more deliberate. If you plan to quit the rat race and reinvent yourself this year, you'll have to speed up the process.

It's never too late. List your immediate goals. Those might include paying off the mortgage, getting an advanced degree or license, securing start-up funds, finding a good location, or learning how to set up a Web site—or just have fun doing the things you love doing.

Now break each goal into a set of near-term action steps. These might include making an extra mortgage payment every six months to own the house twice as fast, or starting the process of applying to the university where you will pursue your advanced education. Near-term actions allow you to closely monitor your progress, so lay out the near-term goals in order and estimate how much time you'll need for each. If you don't know, estimate. You can adjust later. Show the timetable to key members of your support team, especially your inner circle, and revise according to their input. Remember, your closest friends may know more about you than you know about yourself.

Finally, check your progress regularly—every month if your goals are quick, or possibly just twice a year if you have a lot of time. If you fall behind, figure out whether you need to adjust the schedule or redouble your efforts, and if you run into trouble, turn to your support team for advice. Following a plan and staying on schedule will inspire and excite both you and your team members and will give you a growing sense of confidence. Your new career is about much more than just earning a living—it's an opportunity to shed your old life and become exactly who you want to be by working at what you enjoy—and on your own terms.

5

Lifelong Learning Adventures

Former New York Jets quarterback Joe Namath, now in the Hall of Fame, once guaranteed victory in the Super Bowl—and delivered. But it was a different kind of promise that he made to his oldest daughter, Jessica, a few years ago when she had begun to talk about where she intended to go to college and at one point boasted, "I'll be the first to finish college in my family."

"You want to bet?" her famous father shot back.

It turns out that the man known as Broadway Joe for some time had been musing about finishing the college education he interrupted in 1965 to cash in on a then-dazzling $427,000 contract to play in the National Football League. That decision resulted in Namath leaving the University of Alabama one semester shy of earning a degree. Now he was heading back to Tuscaloosa (in spirit; he enrolled in the university's external-degree program) to finish what he had started more than forty years earlier, determined to get his diploma before his daughter got hers.

"I'm a little embarrassed," Namath confided to the *New York*

115

Times. "But everybody keeps telling me it's great, that it might persuade other people to go back to get their degree." Always a leader on the field, Namath was a bit of a follower in the game of life, at least as it relates to education. His return to college no doubt spurred some to follow in his path. But the truth is, men and women have been going back to school in ever larger waves for many years, seeking not so much to show up their young ones as to broaden their own knowledge just for fun, to build new skills, or to pursue long-suppressed though not forgotten dreams and goals.

Adults going back to campus remains an underappreciated trend. Speaking to Katie Couric on NBC's *Today Show*, author Tom Wolfe joked "I could never blend in" on the campuses he visited to research his *I Am Charlotte Simmons*. But Wolfe was wrong. He could have blended in quite easily had he tried. It was just that his research sent him looking for frat boys and sorority girls—not the burgeoning number of Ageless Explorers moving into the nearly one hundred existing or planned communities in the United States linked to universities where adults can and in droves do move in and take classes for fun at little or no charge. Adults are returning to campus around the world, from the University of Barcelona in Spain to the University of Oulu in Finland. These and hundreds more are accepting adult applications in record numbers—not just from their countrymen but also from students around the globe.

A useful Web site for anyone considering going back to school is www.studyabroadlinks.com which can connect you to colleges all over the world.

Learning as Play

Can learning really be fun? Our ancestors certainly thought so. The Latin word for education is *ludus*, which also means "play."

Yet the notion of learning as play or fun would baffle a typical high school student, whose teachers demand that she be on time, have good attendance, memorize facts, hew to authority, and continually compete with others for class rank.

During your primary career years things probably haven't been a lot better than your often oppressive school years. For most of us, learning experiences have been sporadic and mostly governed by outside pressures. Few of us have been in a position to freely pick and choose what and when we wanted to learn. Instead, our jobs often required that we acquire skills that would enable us to be more productive or lead to more rapid advancement. Outside the job, we might have signed up for a fun workshop or two. But continued learning has taken a backseat to raising our families and paying the bills.

Liberated from time-consuming parenting activities and schedules while having more time off from work—extra weeks, months, even years—and driven by your appetite for new ideas and personal growth, education in your power years won't be about getting good grades or pleasing your parents or the boss. It will be about you, about expanding who you are, reigniting your core interests, and maybe even discovering some previously untapped areas of talent or passion. You'll be free to learn exotic languages, study remote cultures or politics, explore new art forms, learn to dance the samba, or rethink your philosophy of God and life.

Traditionally, schools were the exclusive domain of the young, who were packed onto the bus or off to universities to gain the skills they'd need to pursue a fruitful career. By twenty-two or so it was over—your one shot at dedicated learning came to an abrupt end. In that phase of your life, the main purpose of school was to get a diploma and then a degree, which effectively licensed you to compete in the world of work. Then you entered the career stage, braced with all the smarts and skills you thought you'd ever need.

Until just a few decades ago this model worked well enough. Continuing education was largely unnecessary to an agriculture-based or industrial-age workforce. Until the 1950s, most people earned their keep on the assembly line or driving a truck or plowing the fields. Few jobs required more than a high school education. If your parents or grandparents had a need for enhanced work skills, their learning opportunities were usually on-the-job, often in a mentor/apprentice dynamic. And since most careers were built on manual labor, with the speed of innovation modest, learning how to use a plow or slide rule in your youth would probably serve you through your entire work life.

But we are destined to carve out a new role for education. Thanks to our parents' resolve, sacrifice, and commitment, a decades-long economic boom that began in the 1950s, and educational deferments from the military, we went to college in record numbers. In fact, through our initial learning years, education was a priority, and there was a fivefold increase in college enrollment in the United States between 1940 and 1970.

As a college education for the young became the norm, the world began to change. Swiftly evolving technologies began to require new skills and repeated retraining, which you embraced or were left behind to lead a mediocre and unsatisfying life. At the same time, the smaller baby bust generation behind us has been shrinking the target market for traditional educational institutions, which for years had known nothing but growth. To survive, many colleges have been redesigning their programs around the needs of older learners. In addition, to accommodate the busy lives of working men and women, the number of weekend and evening classes and work-site programs have quickly multiplied. For example, aerospace giant Boeing began a work-site learning program in 1990 primarily for younger workers, but today extends learning opportunities to all employees at a wide variety of times and places. The company so values extended learning that it tells all employees they are expected to take an interest in their own development through the lifelong learning opportunities the company offers, including thousands of job-site learning programs in aviation, communications, computing, engineering, math, production, retirement planning, and more. These days the concept of going back to school—or having school come back to you—post-youth is firmly embedded and will continue to blossom in your next stage of life.

In addition, because of the increasing speed of innovation in business, most workers will need to retrain multiple times during their career years. A National Research Council study asserts that a worker's occupational half-life (the span of time it takes for half of a worker's skills to become obsolete) has declined to as few as three years from as many as fourteen in recent decades. Going forward, it is expected that the average worker will hold seven jobs during his or her working life and will therefore require regular retraining.

We heartily recommend taking sabbaticals for extended learning leaves. The idea of a sabbatical is borrowed from agriculture and refers to farmers leaving fields unplanted every seven years to let the soil regenerate. This approach long ago was extended from the farm to the university, where professors commonly take leaves to further their studies or publish a work. Now companies are warming to extended leaves, recognizing them as a way for employees to recharge their intellectual batteries and enhance their job skills in something of a payback for the marathon hours they've been asked to work and the extra years many will need to stay on the job. If we'll be living and working longer, having some lengthy breaks along the way can be rejuvenating.

Currently just 5 percent of U.S. companies grant paid sabbaticals, although 20 percent permit unpaid leaves. The average length of time spent away from work for paid and unpaid sabbatical leaves is five weeks after five years of service. Those who have taken advantage of such programs and the bosses they report to almost universally agree that an extended leave can work wonders on a tired soul.

Michael Olmstead, pastor of University Heights Baptist Church of Springfield, Missouri, had never enjoyed more than a basic vacation in forty years in the ministry. A few years ago he began suffering from severe burnout, a pervasive and little-recognized problem among the clergy. They are on call twenty-four hours a day and spend much of their time with society's less fortunate, which can wear a person down. Olmstead didn't even recognize the extent to which it was getting to him, but one of his parishioners, Wayne, a history professor at nearby South-west Missouri State University, noticed an edginess creeping into Olmstead's manner and felt that his pastor might benefit from some time off. So Wayne organized an effort to fund a three-month sabbatical for Olmstead, who used the time to attend a theological renewal program in the mountains of New Mexico. "It was well worth it," Wayne reflected, adding that after Olmstead returned, "his sermons had a different tone to them." Olmstead says he rediscovered his passion for learning and the excitement of preaching. Now his congregation insists that he take an extended leave for rejuvenation as often as is practical.

The Joy of Being a Student Again

We recognize that there's nothing easy about deciding to hit the books again, whether in short bursts or long stretches. Being a beginner in adulthood can be very disorienting. Barbara Kaden of Point Pleasant, New Jersey, was mortified her first day back at school as an adult. "I hadn't been in a school for almost fifty years and, frankly, I never really enjoyed the classroom," she recalls. But her desire for change and a fresh start drove her to overcome her anxiety. "I had been feeling like I was in a rut, like I had stopped growing," she says. "My world had gotten kind of small. I was spending time with the same people, doing the same things."

Kaden badly needed a spark in her life, and today she laments that it took her so long to find an international learning program for adults. Her first class was in Italy and included eight days in Verona and seven days in Venice. There were lectures and slide shows about art and architecture, Italian history and contemporary Italian life. Her group took daily walking trips to local attractions and had plenty of free time to wander about the local communities. In Venice, she traveled freely on the fabled Grand Canal, interacting with locals and other curious visitors from around the world.

"This incredible experience was far different from the way I remember education," Kaden says. "This was enjoyable and exciting, and the program even helped take my life in a different direction. I am now studying Italian at my community college and learning about Italian art at the library and on the Internet. And I have made many new friends as my learning experiences continue to open up new worlds for me."

More than any previous generation, we have built our lives around information and learning, ultimately coming to the belief that knowledge is more powerful than social class, financial status, or physical prowess. Whereas other generations may have found comfort in the strength of their union, church, or membership club, we are an individualistic and meritocratic generation inclined to believe that ideas and the strength and breadth of our knowledge are more important than any other variable in helping to realize our life dreams.

In 1981, when he was thirty-one, Ken published his second book, titled *Millennium: Glimpses into the 21st Century*, in collaboration with Dr. Alberto Villoldo, with contributions from twenty of the most seminal and sometimes controversial thinkers and philosophers of our era, including Carl Rogers, Karl Pribram, Jean Houston, and Timothy Leary. Jonas Salk supplied a chapter, "The Future of Human Intelligence," in which he proposed that human evolution was at a turning point. Darwin's survival of the fittest was giving way to what Salk called "survival of the wisest." His emerging view—which he shared with Ken and wrote about in *Millennium*—was that information, knowledge, and wisdom would become the world's most precious assets. He believed that boomers, besides being the first generation to benefit from his polio vaccine, would be the first group driven by a lifelong appetite for increasingly sophisticated levels of global knowledge.

Our generation has yet to prove its ultimate mettle in this regard. But there is no doubt that we will approach our power years with the highest levels of formal and informal education ever, and that thanks to the Internet and other easy-access information sources, we'll be able to readily quench our thirst for continual learning in the years ahead. Sociologists note that in its retirement years each generation aspires to do more of what they enjoyed in their youth but didn't have time for as midlife adults. Raised in the shadow of the Depression, our parents had lives that were usually characterized by modest levels of advanced education, hard work, and not much carefree recreation. In their retirement, they have pursued pastimes, housing arrangements, and social dynamics that have allowed them to, in a sense, return to the carefree, playful moments that were in such short supply when they were younger.

For many of us, our college years were both a time for learning and time to have a blast. We spent late nights arguing about philosophy, music, and sexuality; thought-provoking professors challenged our values and beliefs. The excitement that came from building new friendships was based more on intellectual compatibility than on neighborhood proximity. But before we knew it, these years were over and we became fully immersed in our marriages, the lives of our kids, and the incredibly high-pressured modern world of work. Can you imagine that during your power years you will be free once again—this time with a bit more world experience—to ignite those learning engines?

As we argue throughout this book, the linear model of life—childhood, education, career, then retirement and rest—is crumbling. A new, more cyclic culture of lifelong learning is taking root as millions of avid learners enter later life—and as educational institutions, long geared exclusively to young students, begin to notice. To accommodate the coming rush, some universities are even beginning to award credit for life experience. The American College Testing Association recently developed a formal life-experience evaluation that schools are using to award college credits. In lieu of SAT scores and high school transcripts, returning students are asked to provide their personal portfolio, including a presentation of work-related experiences and skills. In short, the world of education has begun to grasp the importance of serving and marketing itself to adults.

But our generation's love of learning is being noticed by more than just traditional educational institutions. Cookware departments at Macy's now offer culinary seminars; cruise lines provide lectures from geologists and religious philosophers on their trips to the Far East; health clubs and gyms provide workshops on health and nutrition; Home Depot runs learning programs on renovating; hospitals provide lectures on self-care; and, of course, the Internet is a portal to nearly everything.

Several years ago, while at the World Economic Forum in Davos, Switzerland, Ken had the good fortune of enjoying a memorable dinner discussion with Sir Tim Berners-Lee, the brilliant scientist who has been credited with inventing the World Wide Web in the late 1980s. Ken asked Berners-Lee (himself a boomer) what his initial intent was in this extraordinary creation. Was it to create a massive new porn industry? A global maze of chat rooms? An at-your-touch airline reservation service? His answer was that he simply had been trying to set up a means by which "everyone could easily share what they knew with anyone who wanted to know it." Information is oxygen for our generation and knowledge is power.

Third-Age Learning: A Worldwide Revolution

Lifetime learning has its strongest roots in Europe and Asia, where populations are growing older sooner than in the United States due to higher life expectancies and lower fertility rates. Europe was the first continent to fully embrace education in maturity, starting in France in 1973, when the Toulouse University of Social Sciences began offering a gerontology course for retirees. This program grew into what is known as a University of the Third Age (U3A), a well-rounded learning experience centered on the interests and schedules of third-age or mature learners. Europeans' interest in adult learning is based on a philosophy about the potential for continued growth and contribution in maturity, from which youth-obsessed Americans have a lot to learn.

After emerging in the 1970s, these European third-age notions spread quickly. In 1981 the British improvised with a new model employing older men and women not just as learners but also as teachers, alternately imparting knowledge they had acquired in their lifetime and soaking up the experiences of others. Today England, Scotland, and Ireland alone have more than two hundred fifty U3As. Membership is nearing fifty thousand. Other countries that have embraced lifetime learning through U3As include Australia, Switzerland, the Netherlands, Italy, Spain, Sweden, Finland, Norway, and Poland.

Asia has a similar network it calls the University of the Aged, and there are more than four hundred outlets that offer studies to half a million adults over age fifty in China and Japan, whose populations are among the oldest in the world. Typical classes include poetry, politics, health, history, calligraphy, music, and dancing as well as broader curricula aimed at improving your life and understanding foreign cultures.

Elderhostel (www.elderhostel.org) is a leader in breaking down the barriers between learning and leisure. Part travel agency, part university, part extreme adventure club, this outfit declares "The World Is Our Classroom" and makes good on the claim. Elderhostel programs take place throughout the world, and the nonprofit institution offers an extraordinary range of classes and programs. In 1975, its first year of operation, Elderhostel had two hundred course enrollments at five sites. Now more than a quarter of a million students participate at nearly two thousand universities, conference centers, parks, museums and cultural institutions in more than a hundred countries. There is no homework, no grades, and no exams. In many instances, Elderhostel creates the ultimate learning experience by allowing participants to live their subject of interest. Course offerings range from watercolor painting in the Catskills forest or Hot Springs desert to glass working at the Corning Museum of Glass or silversmithing in New Mexico.

Elderhostel students range in age from fifty-five to one hundred, and whereas most young people can't wait to leave school for their vacations, Elderhostel students can't wait to attend school for theirs. You live in dormitory rooms, usually when campuses are on summer break, and eat with others in the dining halls. The environment is safe, the rooms and meals are inexpensive, and the social interaction is exhilarating. The instructors enjoy the liveliness of the classes and the high participation rates of students. Professors accustomed to classes with sleepy twenty-year-olds suddenly find themselves confronting seasoned folks willing to challenge conventions, ask penetrating questions, and bring their personal experience to bear on tough issues. Debates that start in a classroom carry over to the dining hall and dorm rooms. In the relaxed yet intellectually charged program atmosphere, students find not only new ideas but also new friends.

You don't just study art from books and lectures at Elder-hostel; you also visit the villages where Monet lived and view his masterworks in Parisian museums. You don't just learn about ecology; you also can camp in the dunes of Baja, California, and trace the migration of gray whales. You don't just listen to music; you also explore America's greatest music, from blues to jazz on a Mississippi River paddleboat traveling between Memphis and New Orleans. You don't just read about history; you also physically retrace the steps of Lewis and Clark. You can learn to paint in Nantucket, fly a hot-air balloon with your grandchildren, join student orchestras, study literature in London, bike the rim of the Grand Canyon, or conduct research to help protect endangered species in the Amazon jungle. Experts join you for lectures and field trips and lively discussions with faculty and fellow participants. All that's needed is an inquiring mind, an adventurous spirit, and being open to learning and discovery.

Charlotte and Harold Feldman from Newton, Massachusetts, have explored the world through Elderhostel activities for twenty years. They have traveled to Alaska to study marine biology and to France for a barge trip, among many others. Originally they weren't so sure the organization was for them. "It'll be all old people," Harold says he figured, laughing about the misconception. "I was wrong. Elderhostel is a wonderful way to go on trips you'd long thought about but never made. And we've made some great new friends."

There are many other choices to consider. In Los Angeles, the PLATO Society (Partners in Learning, Actively Teaching Ourselves) borrows from the British-style U3A by teaching without teachers. "The whole idea is that we teach and learn together," says Alice Bear, a member of the society. "We're not passive students having somebody lecture to us." PLATO discussion groups usually involve fourteen participants, and during a standard fourteen-week term everyone takes a turn as discussion leader. Topics include history, space, political science, classical music, and literature. The leader is responsible for an in-depth look at some aspect of the course topic.

The PLATO Society also hosts guest speakers, often from the University of California at Los Angeles, who may address topics as diverse as pre-Columbian culture and the consideration of God, man, and genetics. Members may audit undergraduate courses at UCLA and participate in special seminars and retreats. "Most of us have been in careers where we haven't had time to study many things, and when we retire, it's a marvelous chance to be students again," says Ruth Gussen, a professor of pathology at UCLA and president of the society.

Your Excellent Learning Adventures

Why keep learning? We believe there are three primary reasons: to discover untapped interests, to hone your skills, and to satisfy your need for personal growth.

1. Discover Untapped Interests

John holds a master's degree in aeronautics from the Massachusetts Institute of Technology and was a lead designer for the Apollo space program. Immediately after retiring, he elected to spend twelve hours a week in a different kind of laboratory: the kitchen classroom at nearby Bristol Community College. There he broadened his technical expertise to include the professional preparation of a poached salmon with hollandaise sauce. John's mission these days is to take control of his kitchen and give his wife time to pursue her career as an artist. He's also having a lot of fun discovering the way good food is put together and creating his own concoctions.

For most, experimenting with new recipes won't necessarily be the answer. But learning something—anything—that interests you can be the key to opening new doors to your own creativity and help you find hobbies and activities that enrich your life. Your career years may have left you in a rut. That's understandable. If you wanted to learn to sculpt or build a sailboat, when would you have had the time? In your next life stage, time will no longer be a barrier.

June Sims of Ada, Oklahoma, started innocently with a basic art course at a nearby college after she retired. "I didn't know a thing about drawing," she recalls. But she pushed through her doubts, and one course led to others—in oils, watercolors, and then pastels. Soon Sims was painting between classes. Then she started winning regional art shows. "I even sold a few pieces," she says. "But that's not why I do it. The work completely occupies me, and I have met wonderful people. Art has given me a whole new life."

Bernard, a former CEO, retired at sixty-two and knew just what he wanted to do next. He enrolled at the Chicago-Kent College of Law. "We thought he was kidding," his daughter, Linda, says. "We didn't believe him until he was in school." Law school had its challenges. "It was a lot harder than I thought," Bernard says. "The last time I was in school was in 1958." But he found that his maturity helped him keep things in perspective in ways that younger students weren't able. Some of them even asked for his counsel when they began cracking under the pressure. Now Bernard is a volunteer at the Legal Assistance Foundation, an agency that offers free legal services to people who can't pay.

After a thirty-year career with the Associated Milk Producers, Phil took a course at the University of Texas to pursue a calling in social work. "I wanted to retire to something, not from something," he says. Now he works with troubled high school students. "Going back to school was challenging," he says. "But I wanted to work with teenagers. How can you find anything more satisfying than helping others? I know I make a difference."

Cliff of Savannah, Georgia, always loved tennis. So when the former sales executive retired, he went to school at the U.S. Tennis Association and today is an accredited tournament umpire working six matches a year. Peg Phillips is a character actress who played the storekeeper Ruth Ann in the quirky television series *Northern Exposure*, has appeared in at least eight movies, and has had guest roles on *Seventh Heaven, Touched by an Angel*, and *E.R.* Phillips didn't start acting until she retired as a tax accountant and then went to the University of Washington drama school at sixty-six.

2. Hone Your Skills

As we've discussed, a lot of us will be working in our later years—for love or money. So we'll want to make sure we're getting the most out of the experience, whether it's a continuation of our primary career or a whole new pursuit. Why not take the time to go back to school and pick up the skills you'll need for a quick jump start or a salary upgrade? And while some will learn new things to enhance their existing skills base, others will use their extended longevity and free time to master a new area of work, craft, or hobby. A newspaper reporter might elect to take courses in fiction writing in preparation for her first attempt at writing a novel. A seasoned business manager might learn a foreign language to better manage his international vendors. A semiretired physician might study new breakthroughs in alternative medicine to recraft his medical practice. Some might even resume their skills—building from a long submerged area of interest.

Ken relates the following story about his mother:

When I was growing up, relatives and friends would often comment that my mom had exceptional talent as a dancer when she was younger. They would rave about her gifts in ballet, tap, samba, and nearly every kind of modern dance form, and they would comment on the various dance troupes and follies that sought her out as a rising star as a teen in Newark, New Jersey, in the 1930s. These stories always amused me, as my mother had given up dancing before I can even remember. She chose to go to work as a manager in my dad's chain of retail clothing stores and stayed with it for decades. I had enjoyed watching my mom dance at a few parties, weddings, and Bar Mitzvahs over the years, and while it was obvious that she was very graceful, I never had much of a sense that dancing had been that big a deal in her life.

Then in 1990, when my parents sold their business and retired to Florida, my mom commented that she really missed the challenge of work and couldn't imagine what she might do with herself now that she had so much free time. Her first two years of retirement were restful but boring. Halfheartedly, I suggested that she return to her tap-dancing studies. Several weeks later, she reported that my suggestion had rung a bell and that she had found a dance studio near her retirement community that offered an evening tap-dance class for beginning-level dancers. It had been more than half a century since she had last tapped, so she bought a new pair of tap shoes and some black leotards. Then, on a quiet Tuesday night in South Florida, seventy-one-year-old Pearl Dychtwald anxiously drove her car to the studio, where her teacher lined her up with sixteen other students, mostly under the age of twelve. The instructor was humored by having this older woman in her class and suggested that she take it very easy with the steps until she had the feel of things again.

As the stereo came alive, it was as though half a century passed in an instant, and my mom performed each step with style and flair. Her classmates and her instructor were amazed. The following Tuesday, the owner of the studio asked if she might teach an advanced-level class. She agreed, but only under the terms that she could also take private lessons from the head of the studio, a top-rated tap dancer. My mom had become a student again as well as a teacher, and she loved it all.

Nearly a year later, I still had never seen my mother perform and surprised her with an unannounced cross-country visit at a recital in which she had an extensive tap solo. During the first hour of the show, I enjoyed the singing and joke-telling of the amateur ensemble, but grew tense as my mom's act neared. Finally, out she soared in her top hat, tuxedo tails, black leotard, and black satin tap shoes and wearing an electrifying smile I had rarely seen. Her performance was graceful and youthful and as she finished, the audience stood for a rousing ovation. I couldn't help but think that Mom had returned to her true calling and found a way to rejuvenate her life.

In the years since, she has come to spend several hours each day teaching tap to kids and seniors and continuing to study the dance form. She has even become a bit of a legend as tappers visiting South Florida seek her out to exchange moves, trade stories, and just have fun. Two years ago, when she required hip replacement surgery, her primary motivation was to dance again. The surgery went well, and Pearl Dychtwald no doubt is tapping up a storm somewhere right now.

3. Satisfy Your Need for Personal Growth

Surveys show that the simple joy of learning tops the list for why adults go back to school. Stripping away subjects and teaching methods that do not interest us, it seems, transforms learning into *ludus*—both education and fun. If you have an innate desire to keep improving, it becomes easier when new pursuits are viewed as play instead of work.

During your hardworking parenting years, your perspectives may have narrowed more than you realize. Now is a perfect time to question your basic assumptions about work, creativity, fun, family, and yourself—and break free from the old habits and mindscapes that may now be boxing you in. In your power years you will have the time to reflect on how you became who you are and to envision who you might become. Remember, the maturing caterpillar doesn't dream of becoming an older, more feeble version of itself—it dreams of transforming into a butterfly. You can transform, too.

Big changes lie ahead: grandchildren, the loss of loved ones and the birth of new relationships, new careers and hobbies, health issues, relocation to new parts of the country or world. Each change presents an opportunity to learn more about who you really are and what you really want; in other words, to continue to grow and develop. The philosopher and psychiatrist Carl Jung held that the task of later life was to explore your full human potential by tapping parts of your personality you had long neglected. If you've been shy and reserved, you can try to be more outgoing. If you've been excessively analytical, you can try to unleash your artistic side. You'll probably find that your previous life experiences have prepared you for these kinds of extensions and expansions at this new point in your life.

Most of us have a story or two about a friend or relative who called it quits too early and has been mentally wasting away for years. While it's generally assumed that most young people dislike older adults and even the aging process—a concept termed "gerontophobia" by Pulitzer Prize–winning author and renowned geriatrician Robert Butler—Ken's work has revealed that it's not necessarily additional birthdays that people worry about. Instead, people dislike the stagnancy that many older people exhibit, and the degree to which some elect to remain so set in their ways and living in the past that they are out of touch.

Instead of giving in to growing old, we're talking about older and still growing! Seen this way, continued learning may very well be the best antiaging medicine available. Losing your mental vitality is a travesty to be avoided at all costs. Your next stage of life will be rife with time and opportunity to learn and grow and keep surprising yourself.

After he retired, Ralph enrolled in the Academy of Lifelong Learning at Trinity College in Connecticut to study ancient Roman architecture. Why? "You reach a point in your life, you gather all these things, a house, a car, then you want to go on and do something more," he says. Richard had a different awakening when he retired. For most of his adult life he had pondered the link between religion and science, often engaging colleagues and family in long discussions on Buddhism, Judaism, and other religions. His long search for answers prompted him to pursue a doctorate in theology at the University of California at Berkeley. He says the experience greatly deepened his sense of purpose and helped quench his thirst for answers.

Mimi started studying literature in her sixties. "I just didn't appreciate the value of Shakespeare in college, when I thought it was a bunch of mumbo jumbo," she says. "Now I can't wait to get to class." John, another adult learner, concurs: "I have a love of learning and wanted an educational experience that provided intellectual stimulation and personal satisfaction." Whereas young people view learning as a means to enhance their careers, says Constance Swank, research director for AARP, "we know from our study that midlife and older adults are looking to enhance their lives."

The World Is Your Classroom

Now you have the freedom to shape and customize your mature education from an expanding variety of resources. The classroom may still play a role. But you will be free to supplement formal instruction with trips and lectures and other, more innovative options. Let's look at four basic choices: third-age universities, virtual learning, experiential learning, and independent study.

1. Third-Age Universities

Pioneering this effort are the hundreds of colleges in the United States that house an Institute for Learning in Retirement (ILR) on campus. For a list go to www.eckerd.edu. Globally, there are hundreds more universities catering to adults through what are known as third-age universities, or U3As. These include top learning institutions in China, Japan, England, Spain, Poland, Canada, Australia, and many other developed nations. The world of U3As can be explored at www.worldu3a.org. Another helpful site is www.mentor.ac, which is run by Mentor International, an international studies consultant with offices in Thailand, England, and the Philippines.

ILRs take many forms. In St. Petersburg, Florida, for example, the Academy of Senior Professionals at Eckerd College (ASPEC) has 350 accomplished members from a wide range of professions and walks of life. These are people who excelled at their careers before retiring and want "to keep creating, keep producing," says Merle Allshouse, former ASPEC director. Members attend lectures and panel discussions on topics from boat-building to opera and discussion groups on topics from science and society to poetry and investing. "The intellectual aspect of the organization was the thing that really got me," says Bob Siver, a former president. "We study right along with the young students. I earned honors in science and economics at the University of Pennsylvania in 1951, but until ASPEC I had little exposure to liberal arts."

Innovative schools are cropping up worldwide to cater to the schedules and learning needs of adults. While many don't offer formal degrees, they do provide valuable instruction in and introductions to just about any subject. The Learning Annex (www.learningannex.com) is North America's largest provider of adult education, offering nearly eight hundred seminars each month in places such as New York, Los Angeles, San Francisco, San Diego, Calgary, Edmonton, Vancouver, and Toronto. Topics include personal growth, business and career opportunities, health and healing, sports and fitness, spirituality, relationships, and high tech.

In Albany, New York, there is Knowledge Network (www .knowledgenetwork.com), which offers more than a hundred classes each month on topics from horseback riding to working with stained glass. In Washington, D.C., there is First Class, which offers seminars on how to plan a walking vacation, Zen, how to quit your job and follow your dreams, wine, and how to sell a movie script. Other adult learning institutions include Discover U in Seattle, Washington (www.discoveru.com), Boston Center for Adult Education in Boston, Massachusetts (www.bcae.org), Learning Exchange in Sacramento, California (www.learning exchange.com), Learning Connection in Providence, Rhode Island (www.learnconnect.com), Colorado Free University in Denver, Colorado (www.freeu.com), and the Learning Studio in Pennsylvania and New Jersey (www.learningstudio.com). Check your telephone directory or the Internet for enticing programs in your area.

2. Virtual Learning

Maybe you want to learn and keep improving but don't want to trudge to class each week. That's the way Clint Stirling of San Antonio, Texas, felt after he retired from the air force and went to work in the tech department of an insurance company. He knew he'd need a new degree to move up the corporate ladder, but he had little interest in returning to a traditional classroom. His solution: pursue a degree in information technology at the University of Phoenix Online (www.phoenix.edu). "I love to do schoolwork from my home, at my convenience," Stirling says. "If I were to attend traditional night school, I would have to drive, park, walk, sit for four hours, walk, drive, and go home at ten o'clock at night and be extremely tired. In my humble opinion, I learn better by applying the information from the text rather than listening to long lectures in a classroom and then testing my rote memory."

Online studies may be the hottest thing to happen to education—ever. Some five hundred thousand classes a year in the United States are now offered via the Web, often from accredited bricks-and-mortar universities that recognize Internet studies for formal degrees. Originally geared to young students adept at navigating the Net, virtual classwork has emerged as extremely well suited for those adult learners who are not seeking live interpersonal contact and appreciate the convenience of having their computer serve as a portal for educational adventure.

Daily lectures can be downloaded when convenient, and most research can be done over the Net. Students have access to class notes as well as prominent lecturers and unusual courses online that are unlike anything available at a community college. Most classes are "independent start," where students "go" to class at their convenience. But others are "group start," where classes start at a specific time and students are expected to attend online and on time.

A great place to examine the possibilities is at www.life longlearning.com. This Web site lists online schools, their courses and degrees, and what they cost. It also lists how course work at each institution can be accessed, including by radio, audio- or videocassette, cable or satellite TV, CD-ROM, or the Web. Other helpful Web sites include www.petersons.com, www.geteducated.com, and www.distance.gradschools.com.

If you have a favorite university, try logging on to its Web site (usually the home page is the name of the school with .edu at the end—for example, www.columbia.edu or www.stanford.edu). Many of them now have online universities and will offer a demonstration upon inquiry. Universities throughout the world are jumping on this bandwagon, from the University of Victoria in British Columbia, Canada (www.uvcs.uvic.ca), to the University of Auckland in New Zealand (www.auckland.ac.nz).

3. Experiential Learning

Increasingly, leisure and education are merging at a nexus known as experiential learning, essentially the creative combination of fun and learning through doing. Forget about passive travel, poolside bingo, or mindless TV viewing. You can absorb history while vacationing in ancient cities and towns, study environmental science while on spectacular mountain hikes and ocean cruises, and immerse yourself in the arts not by reading about painting and sculpture but by visiting the capitals of artistic achievement.

In addition to the impressive Elderhostel activities we've discussed, there are numerous terrific programs available to adults interested in experiential learning. World Explorer Cruises (www.wecruise.com) ripped out its casino to make room for a library that enhances the historical and cultural aspects of the regions where it sails. "We are not just about the ship; we are about the places we visit," explains Kristina Nemeth, the company's program manager. The ship spends summer months in and around Alaska and winter months in and around Central America. Packages include sixteen hours of lectures on history, anthropology, biology, and geology. Sample titles include: Glaciers: Alaska's Ice Monsters, The Wreck of the *Exxon Valdez*: The Aftermath, and Heroes and Villains of the Alaskan Gold Rush. There are also lectures and trips ashore. Each trip also features an Artist-in-Residence Program with painting, dancing, storytelling, and carving instruction from guest experts. In its library, World Explorer Cruises has an extensive Alaska Collection as part of its sixteen thousand books, the largest library afloat.

Some towns with high densities of retirees are turning their entire community's culture into learning environments. In Palm Beach, thousands of members of the Society of the Four Arts are treated to exhibits and concerts with fellow enthusiasts of art, music, drama, and literature. The society attracts all manner of artists, from those who work with watercolors to others expert in Chinese sculpture. It has concert pianists and flamenco dancers. Visit their Web site at www.fourarts.org and have your mind expanded with the wide range of lectures, films, exhibits, classes, and activities provided to retirees everywhere in their community.

For people with other ideas of fun and learning, there is the exploding world of fantasy camps for adults that we explored in chapter 3. Themes run the gamut of crafts, dance, photography, religious study, cooking, and flying. Camp Mom, a retreat in the San Gabriel Mountains an hour north of Los Angeles, has the attractive motto "No Kids, No Men, No Makeup, No Stress, No Cooking." A weekend of good food, stress-free lodging, and enjoyable lifestyle-related classes at Camp Mom costs just $219. "The food is great because you don't have to plan it, think about it, or do the dishes," says Denise Hatch, who has attended the camp four times. "You just show up." For a more traditional camp experience, Camp Cheerio, run out of High Point, North

Carolina, offers summer programs for fifty-plus campers who want to rediscover canoeing, archery, and rifles.

4. Independent Study

You won't need a formal program to keep learning. In your next stage of life you can do it through the libraries, museums, art galleries, parks, social clubs, religious institutions, alumni organizations, periodicals, and instructional CDs and videos you may already know so well. All that is required is imagination and initiative. You can attend lectures at nature centers or zoos, participate in music, dance, or theater, take a part-time job, or join a political or nonprofit group. Or you can contract for private lessons of any sort. Maybe you'd like to learn how to make your own clothes; there are hundreds of seamstresses who would mentor you if you paid them for their time. If you'd like to learn to write a novel, you can readily retain an English teacher or professor—or a local author—to give you some tips. The same goes for learning to surf the Internet, improve your golf swing, or master Mandarin. Virtually all communities have talented resources for hire.

Richard, a retired math professor, is a model of independent study. He designs Web pages and has learned by doing with support from books such as *HTML for Dummies*. Richard is also learning Russian on his own. "When I was much younger there were no computers," he says. "Now I can study Russian by reading Russian newspapers on the Internet. I exchange e-mail with people in Russia. I listen to radio broadcasts from Russia over the Internet, recording them on tape, then listening to them while exercising." He takes extended trips to Russia, where he stays with Russian families and volunteers as an English teacher.

Katherine has blended classroom learning with independent study. At fifty-four she went to Washington University in St.

Louis to earn a master's degree in teaching. Then she lived in Europe, learning French, and attending the University of Paris. She joined the Peace Corps, studied rural community development at the University of Maryland, and taught in Fiji at the University of the South Pacific. Now she works with foreign students at the Webster Grove Nature Study Society. She studies gardening at the Botanical Gardens in St. Louis and uses her knowledge to design flower arrangements for the library at Webster University.

Join the Revolution

How do you get started? Reflection sounds wonderful. But, as we've noted, most of us haven't had a lot of time to visit the mountaintop lately. Can you just push a button and be on your way? Probably not. But rest assured that you'll have ample resources to guide you as you fashion a later-life curriculum suited to your individual needs. Here are some simple steps to help you get started:

1. Establish Your New Learning Hopes and Goals

Think back to when you selected a major in college. Of course, the decision may have been misguided, and you may have switched majors several times before lighting on one that seemed right. Today you know far more about yourself. While choosing a path is rarely easy, the pressure is off because you can do what you want versus what other people expect of you, and you won't be encumbered by having to make a decision upon which your entire lifetime economics and happiness are resting. In earlier chapters we reflected on what would help us identify a new career or hobby. We can apply some of those same lessons to continuing education and the quest for continued personal growth.

Think about things that have excited you through your life. Have you enjoyed tinkering with mechanical devices, listening to music, writing poetry, coaching your kid's basketball team, taking dancing lessons, teaching at your church, leading a military unit, explaining things to people, providing help to those in need, or reading books? Also, think about activities or fields of interest that you never pursued but that you might find interesting now. Nutrition and health? Mentoring young workers? Writing short stories? Being a radio commentator? Directing a documentary film? Serving as a museum curator? Understanding star patterns? Yoga, Tai Chi, Pilates? It's of utmost importance that you set yourself free to explore what you would now like to learn more about—realizing that it could be a continuation of a previous pursuit or an entirely new area of interest. Then consider what new information or skills would help you pursue this calling. This exercise need not be overwhelming. If travel is your ambition, you might begin by taking a course in foreign culture or religion, or learn a foreign language before setting sail. If you're thinking of starting a small business, maybe you need better management or sales skills. Would a refresher course in accounting help? What about a new or advanced degree, or a brokerage or real-estate license?

Learning also can help expand your network of relationships. What kinds of people would you like to meet? Certainly there are classes or programs that will get you involved with your target type right away, whether it be artists, writers, hikers, bikers, samba dancers, sailors, or political activists.

2. Write Down Your Ideas and Hopes

How many times have you gone to the grocery store with a mental list of six or seven items needed for a recipe and returned home to find that somehow you had forgotten one of the items? That can't happen if you make a list and stick to it. But writing it down does more than give you a crib sheet. The act of putting words on paper helps to sear those words into your consciousness to the point where once you have written it down you often no longer need the mental list. You simply remember better and can more easily focus on anything you have put on paper.

Writing it down also lets you more readily survey your thoughts and recognize shortcomings or redundancies. You get a bigger picture; you can more easily organize your thoughts. This method best allows you to think through all of your goals and match them to areas of learning that will help you reach those goals.

3. Create a Personal Master Plan

In your school days, at the outset of each semester you were given a syllabus outlining what would be covered in each course, when and how you'd be tested, and the books and other resources that would be available. In your next stage of life, such regimens will not exist. Learning during your power years is a choice. You can make it whatever you want, and you should embrace the opportunity to craft a personal learning program that is just right for your needs, rhythms, and ambitions.

A lot of folks will be tempted to wing it. After all, you won't be getting graded, and in most cases your livelihood will not depend on success in your new learning endeavors. But again, it's a good idea to put something on paper. Mastering a new subject or skill can be challenging and frustrating. Having a strategy and game plan will keep you on track. Start with a mission statement, as you did in chapter 4 while preparing for a mature career. This statement should be short and direct, and it should reflect what you want to learn and how you want to use your newly acquired knowledge. Examples of mission statements might be:

I will meet interesting new people and deepen my understanding of foreign cultures by mastering French and then visiting Paris.

I will give back to my community by earning a teaching degree and working in the public schools.

I will improve my writing skills by taking three workshops during the next nine months.

I will attempt to learn an entirely new sport, such as skiing, swimming, or kayaking—even if I'm not very good at it at first.

I will seek a deeper relationship with God and become more at peace with myself by studying the Scriptures.

You won't be starting from scratch. The things you've experienced and learned over a lifetime provide blueprints for what you'll want to learn as you go forward. Reflecting on your personal stockpile of knowledge and experiences gives you an understanding of what you most enjoy and value and what types of learning experiences in the past have been most rewarding. Sometimes learning goals emerge naturally; at other times they emerge only after taking a few wrong turns. So leave plenty of time to settle on the right course of action.

4. Take It in Doable, Bite-Size Steps

Set a realistic timeline for reaching your ultimate goal; get there by breaking down the mission into manageable tasks with interim goals and deadlines. Becoming a chef may seem daunting—but learning about ingredients, preparation techniques, and cooking tools, and mastering one recipe at a time make the process enjoyable. Think about how to combine class work, field work, and independent study for the best overall experience. And don't be shy about asking for feedback from friends who can offer an important reality check on your expectations.

Measure your progress to stay on track. If your goal is to learn chess, schedule a monthly match with a challenging opponent. If your goal is learning the language of HTML, try to build increasingly more sophisticated Web sites every few months. If you're not learning as fast as you'd like, find other resources. That might mean switching classes or hiring a private tutor.

5. Build on Small Wins

Few things are more motivating than success along the way. Even if you enjoy learning, tangible rewards can keep you focused and make it easier to work through the inevitable frustrations. So plan a trip to Napa after making progress in your quest to become a wine expert, or spring for tickets to a concert if you're studying music and have just mastered a difficult piece. To keep momentum, plan your next learning adventure before finishing the first.

As you enter your next stage of life, the pace of educational innovation for people like you will only accelerate. Simple demographics dictate that learning institutions of every sort, from vocational schools to universities, will have no choice but to court and serve you as you seek new knowledge, skills, or even new degrees. In the years ahead, you can expect a whole new spectrum of offerings that will enable you to learn what you want, where you want, and how you want. Watch as free universities, golf, tennis, and race-car driving schools, fantasy sports camps, floating campuses, worksite-based career reinvention centers, Internet universities, and crafts clubs multiply beyond your imagination.

Learning opens the door to new activities and helps you meet interesting people and, ultimately, to better understand yourself. Thinking about lifelong learning now—even before you reach later life—will prepare you for when the time comes and ensure that you make the most of this liberating period just ahead.

6

Where and How to Live

As we inexorably near the age when our parents retired, a dynamic mini-industry of newsletters, books, magazines, and Web sites is blossoming to steer us toward our very own version of real-estate nirvana. We're a mobile generation, more so every day. A Del Webb survey shows that 59 percent of boomers plan to move after quitting their primary careers. That's up from 31 percent in 1999. And 10 percent are also planning to buy a second home.

These figures reflect a restlessness and appetite for lifestyle change our parents didn't possess. Having grown up in rented quarters or living with extended family, many worked hard and spent frugally to get the resources to buy a place all their own. Most weren't about to dump it for something as whimsical as better weather or a view. The relative few who thought that way quickly concluded that if they could afford it, a golf course in Florida or Arizona was where they'd like to end up.

That was then. Today, home ownership is at record highs, but we won't cling to our homes the way Mom and Dad may have. If our kids are destined to move away and our friends disperse, what's keeping us from picking up stakes and looking for something better? Of the folks currently contemplating a retirement relocation, more than half say they will move at least three hours away.

In the United States that probably means moving to another state. In the Del Webb survey, top preferences for our generation in the United States were Florida (21 percent) and Arizona (18 percent) topping the list, followed by North Carolina (10 percent), South Carolina (10 percent), Tennessee (9 percent), Texas (7 percent), Colorado (7 percent), Virginia (7 percent), California (6 percent), New Mexico (6 percent), Georgia (5 percent), New York (4 percent), Kentucky (3 percent), and Pennsylvania (3 percent). Even cold Wisconsin (2 percent) and Maine (2 percent) hold some allure. These diverse results suggest that since many of us have made our living on the road and have already relocated once or twice or more for career or family reasons, we're far less concerned about staying put than any previous generation.

Internationally, surveys show there are plenty of great places to live outside the United States. For example, Sweden and Venezuela are beautiful countries with relatively low costs of living, and, for people who concern themselves with such things, some of the most attractive people on the planet. Meanwhile, Finland, Norway, Canada, Sweden, Switzerland, New Zealand, and Australia are rated as the cleanest countries on earth. Luxembourg, Norway, Denmark, Iceland, and Canada are among the wealthiest nations per capita.

The United States is home to far and away the most computers and computer users. But Japan, Germany, England, France, Italy, and Canada are also big players on the Internet. Countries deemed to have the highest quality of life include Norway, Sweden, Canada, Belgium, and Australia. If travel is important consider that Brazil and Canada rate highly for access to airports, and when it comes to continuing your education, no country provides more choices than India, home to a staggering 8,407 universities—the most in the world.

Ageless Explorers have already begun to scour the map for a particular blend of opportunities suited for them, and they are willing to go anywhere to get it right. Tax rates, crime rates, housing prices, cost of living, weather, cultural attractions, educational opportunities, ease of travel, leisure activities, and interesting job possibilities are all in the mix. This quest for the perfect place to live has given rise to growing media coverage seeking to help us choose the right city or town—or country. *Money* magazine has its annual "best places to retire" feature, and it sponsors a comprehensive and interactive Web site (www.money.com) with a cost-of-living calculator, comparative real-estate values, and both a quick-look and an in-depth analysis of regions to guide us to an idyllic late-life homestead.

Another useful interactive Web site is www.findyourspot .com, which factors in forty criteria to match your needs with a postcareer haven. At www.bestplaces.net you can throw into the mix such criteria as the unemployment rate and expected job growth—not of much concern to yesterday's retiree but something we in our power years may find useful. *Where to Retire* magazine is published six times a year, and there's always a handful of books in print on the subject as well as regionally focused Web sites.

These resources are useful starting points, but don't take them to the bank. In our view, the biggest lapse in the media's guidance is that it centers too much on yesterday's model of retirement. Most of us aren't seeking a pasture to be set out to or for a place to kick up our heels and sip on a mai tai for twenty or more years. We have way too much energy for that. Instead, we're taking stock of what matters most to us now, and when the time comes, we'll go wherever we choose to surround ourselves with the kind of people we enjoy and a climate that suits our bones. We'll be going back to school and looking for opportunities to cycle in and out of jobs we enjoy. We'll be scouting out places that offer the right kind of fitness and volunteer activities as well as recreational and cultural opportunities and the chance to forge new friendships and rekindle or find new intimacies. And if we want to start our own business, things such as the availability of capital and mentors may become important.

We see five major relocation choices taking shape as we move from our primary career years into our power years, and we'll talk about them now.

Should I Stay or Should I Go?

The Del Webb survey makes it clear that many of us will seek out new quarters in our next life stage—some 59 percent of us. Here's how that breaks down: 26 percent say they will stay put for a few years after quitting work and then move; 24 percent say they will move a few years before they retire with the intent of making their new residence the one they'll retire in; and 9 percent say they will move as soon as they retire.

Implicit in all of this: a very large number—41 percent of the boomer generation—say they won't go anywhere. They are people such as Dr. Robert Conn, a cardiologist in Kansas City, Missouri. He quit his practice in 1998 and instead of moving to a Florida golf course stayed in Kansas City, where he continues practicing medicine on a greatly reduced schedule. "I still do what I like most in life, which is practice medicine, and then have a half day to do my thing, whether it's being with grandchildren, working out, or fixing golf clubs for family and friends," Dr. Conn says. His family in the Kansas City area includes a wife and children and three of his and his wife's four parents who are still living. These relationships are a big reason why Conn doesn't wish to leave. He's also having fun working back in the emergency room now that he's more selective with his hours.

In general, those of us who choose to stay put later in our power years will do so because, like Dr. Conn, we'll have managed to cultivate close friends, keep our families nearby, or want to stay with our employer (perhaps in a reduced capacity) to bridge our primary career years to when we'll truly stop working sometime downstream.

As we shift to our next life stage, many of our communities will change along with us. In Stowe, Massachusetts, town fathers are converting the Pompositticut School building into a combination fire station and activities center. The school building, nicely situated near the center of town, became obsolete when another school building was renovated and enlarged while the demand for retiree-oriented recreation was growing. This type of thing will occur repeatedly as our children—the force behind a massive school building wave during the past twenty years—graduate and leave all that brick and mortar idle.

If you decide to stay put, you can rediscover your community and learn about things you may never have had time to appreciate as active parents or career-focused professionals: museums and other cultural and leisure attractions; church groups to help you rediscover your faith and strike up new relationships; local charities and civic organizations to allow you to give something back; and mentors' groups to help you stay busy and relevant. You'll enjoy many of the benefits of moving—new discoveries, pursuits, and relationships—without the drama of uprooting.

Far too much emphasis has been placed on the financial and infrastructure burdens we will place on the system as we reach maturity. Not nearly enough attention has been paid to our potential to change society for the better by staying involved—becoming, say, a foster grandparent, teaching assistant at a local school, or small-business mentor. "We need to uphold and develop the option for public service (in later life) that constitutes the greatest potential 'win-win' combination for individuals and society," writes Marc Freedman in his seminal book *Prime Time*.

Freedman describes neighborhood medical clinics run by retired volunteer physicians and similar efforts by retired volunteer lawyers. What our communities lack today is broad support for retirees who want to give something back. But that will change as we retread and reinvent instead of retire. Volunteerism and other forms of active engagement, Freedman writes, are the keys to "bringing about the kind of transformation that could help revitalize our communities and inject new meaning into later life."

Remaking Our Homes

Whether we stay put or move in our next stage, one thing we'll do in a big way is remake our homes. We anticipate an explosion in remodeling over the next twenty years that will make runaway winners of stocks of companies such as Home Depot and Lowe's as well as homebuilders such as Toll Brothers, Centex, Lennar, and Pulte (which recently acquired the retirement housing innovator Del Webb). Why the expected crush of remodeling? Our generation likes change, and we also want our homes to match our evolving lifestyles. "What I'm seeing now is a lot different than we saw with baby boomers' parents" says Jim Gillespie, CEO of real-estate giant Coldwell Banker. "They didn't want to move, or if they did, it was to a smaller house. Boomers are looking to retire where they enjoy the culture, and to a bigger house than Mom or Dad ever considered."

Our parents tended to accept things the way they were and made the most of it—not us. When we were in college we changed majors and often roommates; later, half of us changed spouses. We've changed jobs and have even changed our workplace, becoming telecommuters, chucking the tie and suit, and wearing jeans on Friday. We are comfortable with change; we even crave it. We understand that, like the computerized Sims game, everything about a house is changeable, and in our power years we'll adapt our surroundings to our evolving wants and needs. How better to get a fresh start after empty nesting, retiring, or a divorce than by remaking the house?

Many of us have already redesigned our kitchens into palatial playrooms to stay close to our hungry, TV-watching teenagers. The oversized kitchen also lets us marry our inner gourmet with our love of entertaining. For twenty years we set up house around family. But as empty nesters we'll have a whole new range of amenities to crave. We'll want home offices and the latest in electronics so we can make the most of home-based part-time work, and many will want mini-gymnasiums to stay physically fit.

For twenty-one years, the two-story Minnesota farmhouse of Jackie and Dean Smith was perfectly suited for family life—three spacious bedrooms and a barn where daughter Darcy showed horses. They had three dogs and a huge garden of ribbon-winning vegetables. But then Darcy left, and maintaining their beloved 1880s home just didn't seem worth it. "We figured we'd been there, we'd done that," says Jackie. The couple wasted little time, moving to a detached town house in Plymouth, Minnesota, where they can walk downtown and still have enough garden space for a few tomatoes and herbs. Their new home is family-friendly, with a community pool often used by their granddaughter Lindsey. But they gutted and remodeled it with themselves in mind. "We looked at what we had and said, 'How are we going to live in it?'" Jackie recalls. They updated the kitchen and went from three bedrooms to two, with one of the original bedrooms functioning as a home office, and they put in a large master bathroom.

While some people seek to downsize, others are upsizing. Mike Tweddle of suburban Detroit recently retired and began building an eight-thousand-square-foot home. "Building this home has been a retirement project for me," Tweddle reflects. "We wanted to put more of our living space on one floor and create space for entertaining and bedrooms for when the kids visit." He and his wife have five children and four grandchildren. The main floor of their new home includes a great room, formal dining room, kitchen with eat-in area, library/media center/office, master bedroom suite and bath, and laundry room. On the lower-level walkout, there are three guest bedroom suites, an exercise room that can be converted to a fourth bedroom, and a room with bar, TV, and karaoke.

There are no best places or standard ways to stay put. Some of us love San Diego, while others prefer Toronto or Rome. Count your blessings if you can afford to stay in a home and community you love. You're doubly blessed if where you want to stay put has low taxes, good medical facilities, cultural attractions, a low crime rate, a low cost of living, flexible job opportunities for adults, and nearby airports—in short, the kind of place that others seek out when searching for their personal nirvana.

Some people will seek to live in the same general area but will dramatically shift their kind of housing. For example, for Max and Kay Schroeder, who had spent their lives in Houston, where Max worked as an advertising executive, the answer was close to home. After considering options near and far, and even musing about life in Tuscany, they settled on a sun-baked region of Texas known as "Texcany" for its rolling landscape similar to the Tuscan hills of Italy. "How could we help but fall in love with it?" says Kay of her new power years home near Wimberley, Texas, between San Antonio and Austin. "This property had such great views and wonderful oak and elm trees all over. And there are lots of wildflowers." The thrill of moving from the city to a sprawling rural setting reenergized them both. "It's the type of place where you wave at the people you see whether you know them or not," Max said, adding that his house is "quiet without being isolated." Max has taken up writing fiction and just published his first novel. Wimberley's thriving art community revived Kay's interest in painting. "I'm an outdoor person," Kay said. "I hate to be closed in. The back of the house is all glass, so when you're inside you feel like you're outside."

Theme Communities

Remember the sixties? Okay, some of us were too young and missed it. Others of us were present but have, well, forgotten a thing or two. Still, most of us will recall the establishment-rattling advent of hippie communes. Whatever went on inside those funky, tie-dyed walls illuminated by scented candles and Lava lamps is not the point. Communes were, at the core, a group of individuals living in one another's company to enjoy the support of a group in an environment they collectively controlled. The smoke and Lava lamps are gone for good, we hope. But in our power years, communal living will make a comeback.

We're not necessarily talking about the kind of institutional communal living many of our parents and grandparents know so well: the old-folks' home, assisted living complex, or nursing home, where you essentially rent quarters and live among strangers of similar age, health, and wealth, and by a set of rules you do not control. The communes of our future, like the locations where we put them, will be carefully thought through for the perfect mix of companionship, stimulation, and convenience. Some will be vast complexes set up by developers for hundreds of people with an interest in gardening, fitness, Zen, or the arts. Others will consist of just three or four friends who want to live with people they love being with.

The possibilities are endless. Already, theme communities have sprouted up for gay men and lesbians, for specific ethnic groups, for those who want a southern lifestyle, and for retired military officers. Sunset Hall in Los Angeles bills itself as a "home for freethinking elders." The ElderSpirit is a residence for artists in Manhattan. At the Wilderness Lake Preserve in Land O' Lakes, Florida, you can get a deep-woods feel, passing a ranger station on the way in and cooling off in the swimming hole instead of a pool. At Bison Ranch (www.bisonranch.net) in Overgaard, Arizona, you can live like a cowboy, including cookouts and lots of horseback riding.

Bison Ranch was just what Christine and Burt Marcus were looking for. Burt is a retired dentist who left his practice and his 107-horse ranch near Albany, New York, several years ago. "When we saw Bison Ranch we fell in love with it," Burt says. "We really enjoy the beauty of all the hills and pine trees. The town is a replica of an old western village, which is important to us because we have two horses. You can even join a posse, which is a real group that rides out and looks for tourists to rescue from the desert." Christine enjoys golf and horseback riding, and they both love to take part in the annual Prada del Sol parade, which features thirteen hundred horses, the biggest horse parade in the world. "We really never retired," Burt says. "We just changed our lifestyle. Christine doesn't let me use the R word."

Jack and Elina Wilson love Bison Ranch for another reason. Both are avid four-wheelers and make use the area's ample woodlands and trails. "We ride our ATVs all over," says Elina. "It's a blast to go out in the woods and go buzzing everywhere with our neighbors and kids."

We know of many women in their fifties—some working and some not—who are already crafting fallback plans. They understand that women live longer than men. They don't want to get caught unprepared and have begun to muse about what might be if they suddenly find themselves alone. Even those who weren't hippies in the sixties recall the excitement and camaraderie of dormitory life. They like the idea of family-style dining and late-night discussions. Maybe four of them will buy a Manhattan co-op or a farm in Alberta, a town house in Berkeley or a house in the south of France, and rehab it to suit their lives—separate entrances, kitchens, and bedrooms, but a spacious common room and dining room for entertaining and each other's evening company when they choose. They might bring in a cook and cleaner or a hair stylist or masseuse or masseur and pool the expense. It would be their house, their way, and so much better than winding up at disparate assisted living centers.

The idea of communal living has plenty of appeal—if we do it as they did on the TV comedies *Friends, Seinfeld, Will and Grace*, or *The Golden Girls*. One of the great attractions of setting up our own commune is that we can place it anywhere we like, from Hawaii to Spain to India, and live among people—both in the community and within our walls—of varying ages and interests to spice life with a bit of the unexpected. Boomers do not want to be isolated from the world. In the Del Webb survey, 75 percent of those who say they will relocate say they want to go someplace with a mix of ages. Only 7 percent said they preferred a community composed entirely of people fifty-five and up—and that figure is a marked falloff from 15 percent in earlier studies.

Curiously, the kind of person seeking no-youth-allowed retirement communities has flip-flopped in recent decades. For our parents' generation, the folks who sought them out tended to be high-income earners. Among boomers, the high-income earners are turned off by these communities; they're not interested in spending decades removed from the laughter of children or spending too much time focused on aches and pains, with everyone the same age and ethnicity. However, the low-income-earning boomers are beginning to seek these communities in droves.

What interests might influence your housing and community preferences? Here are a few themes, and a few ideas on where and how to set up your power years living space:

Health. We are the most health-conscious (though not necessarily the most healthy) generation in history. We stopped smoking and started counting carbs. We made billion-dollar companies of fitness clubs such as Bally's, vitamin marketers such as GNC, and health-food chains such as Whole Foods. Yes, plenty of us are overweight. But with modern medicine, liposuction, and plastic surgery, it's getting easier to look good and feel good into late life, and a large segment of us will dedicate our postcareer years to being more fit than a runway model and (in our minds, anyway) just as sexy. Inevitably, some communities will take up the mission and present themselves as committed to healthy living and all it implies, and we will find them.

Richard Dugas, CEO of Pulte Homes, is counting on it. His research shows that a state-of-the-art fitness center is among the top priorities of folks over age fifty-five moving into one of his company's communities. Also high on the list are all sorts of amenities, such as security guards and a lifestyle manager who arranges parties, trips, and other outings. Today's buyers want smaller houses but with more features such as ample counter space, big cabinets, and large common rooms. But for a great many, nothing trumps a fitness room. "You'd be amazed how many are banging the door down at five-thirty in the morning to get into the fitness club," Dugas says. "Their day doesn't begin until they've worked their muscles."

Leisure and recreation. No question about it, as we've seen, play and fun will be a big part of our power years, and for many of us it will be the most important part. Even if we're logging half days in the E.R., like Dr. Conn, we may value living near or on a golf course or a well-stocked trout stream. If your idea of having fun includes a lot of travel, then you'll want to be near an airport. If cultural attractions and fine dining matter, you can choose to be near a large or hip city. You can always fly to the mountains to ski or rock-climb—unless you want to do it all the time.

For the great outdoors, consider St. George, Utah, in the state's southwestern corner and known as "color country"; it is marked, as *Money* describes it, by "red rocks, deep blue sky, snow-capped mountains in the distance. Just minutes from Snow Canyon and about two hours from Zion National Park, the Grand Canyon and Bryce Canyon. . . . This town is a Mecca for active retirees." It has thirty-five thousand miles of walking trails. Dixie State College is there, providing opportunities for lectures and other cultural events, as well as continuing education. Las Vegas is an easy drive.

Another hiker haven is Roanoke, Virginia, resting in a valley surrounded by the Blue Ridge and Allegheny Mountains and near the Appalachian Trail. Boulder, Colorado, is tough to beat for vistas and outdoor action, including hundreds of miles of biking and hiking trails.

On the pricier side, California's terrific Napa-Sonoma region blends cycling and hiking opportunities with a wide range of winery-based cultural activities. It is just one hour from high culture in San Francisco and three hours from skiing and gambling around Lake Tahoe in the Sierra Nevada.

For plain old fun in the sun you might want to look into Sarasota, Florida, which is considerably less expensive and stereotypical than other cities in the state. Plenty of families of all ages settle there, giving the city a well-rounded age profile. On the Gulf of Mexico, Sarasota has thirty-five miles of beach with flourlike sand. Many homes are on small canals with docks. You can actually get around some neighborhoods in a boat. For a bit more solitude in the Florida sun, the state's northern region has generally been overlooked by folks fleeing the four seasons. Steinhatchee, Havana, and Lynn Haven are blessed with many off-the-beaten-path features, such as a quaint post office and some of the best trout fishing in the United States.

Outside the States, Brazil's Santa Catarina Island is a bargain. The beaches are uncrowded and the small towns that dot the island are colonial and picturesque. Called Floripa by the locals, it's a two-hundred-square-mile island just off the coast of southern Brazil. There are forty-nine major beaches, countless small ones, and dozens of lovely towns, while the nearby city of Florianópolis is large enough to provide all the necessities of life. For a different take, consider lovely, rugged Nova Scotia, Canada, which is especially suited to those seeking a colder climate for things such as ice fishing and skiing and, for transplanting Americans, has the advantage of feeling right at home.

If the arts are your thing, consider Ashland, Oregon, which is home to the 175-acre campus of Southern Oregon University and the renowned Oregon Shakespeare Festival. The state has no sales tax, and it has abundant outdoor pursuits in the shadow of picturesque mountains. "I can catch a steelhead in the river or a trout in the lakes, come home and garden in the afternoon and go to a nice restaurant and a show at night," comments Gary Farnham, a retired physician. The town boasts funky coffee shops and natural-food cafés along with gourmet food shops catering to tourists near Ashland's center, where sit the Oregon Shakespeare Festival's three theaters. Ashland has drawn Shakespeare lovers since the festival was founded in 1935. The city has one of North America's largest classical repertory theater companies with a season that runs from March through October.

Efficient living. For many of us, economics and convenience will be the biggest factors in choosing where to live. We'll be most concerned with stretching the value of our dollars, staying close to loved ones, feeling safe and secure in our homes, and confident in the quality of the available medical care. Fortunately, such places are not all that difficult to find. How can we research them?

The local chamber of commerce can be a great source of information. So, too, is the town clerk in many smaller communities. Real-estate agents who have worked an area for many years can tell you just about anything you want to know. Be sure to ask what types of special services exist to help launch a small business (lenders, mentors) or if any employers in town value mature workers and have innovative programs to woo them. We don't have to travel to do all this research. Libraries in many towns subscribe to out-of-town newspapers, and, of course, the Internet is an invaluable tool.

After settling on a few likely towns, subscribe to the local paper and read it regularly to really get a feel for the place. Is the mayor a jerk? If so, you won't like the people who elected him. Does the town cater to developers? If so, it may grow too fast and lose that friendly feel before our time is up. This is a great way to research real-estate prices. And scouring the classified ads can give you many insights. Help-wanted ads give an idea of local wages, good information whether you're looking for part-time work—or to hire help for your small business or just to cut the lawn. If you're a sports junkie, you may even want to follow the local teams in the paper to see if they are good enough to pack in crowds that generate a lot of excitement. Most of this information is also available on the Internet, where many local papers post an online version. And virtually every chamber of commerce has a Web site.

In general, you'll probably want to focus on a handful of considerations: safety (That's where the crime rate comes in.); affordability (How much are property and income taxes? How much can we earn in a part-time job? How much will we pay for needed services?); medical care (How's the hospital? Are doctors accepting new patients? Will your health plan work there?); climate (It's a short boating season in Maine.); friends and family (Are you close enough to loved ones to stay in touch? Can you find new friends of common interests?); transportation (Where's the airport? Are there enough buses and taxis?); and jobs or volunteer work (What's available? Do employers have flextime and job-sharing opportunities? Will they welcome you as a volunteer in the state park or at the local Red Cross?).

So where are these kinds of communities? Safe, reasonably priced, and engaging are at the core of many studies and guides on retirement living. Some of the best research has been done by John Howells, whose book *Where to Retire* is in its fifth edition. Another winner is *America's Best Low-Tax Retirement Towns* by Eve Evans and Richard Fox. There are literally hundreds of communities to sift through. These are some of our favorites:

- *Savannah, Georgia.* This gentle southern city has a relatively young population to keep life interesting, a warm climate, and tons of history. Modest homes go for $200,000.

- *Franklin, Tennessee.* This is another town where folks of all ages tend to settle, not just visit. The population is relatively young. It, too, has plenty of southern history, with a Victorian downtown district that's listed on the National Register of Historic places. Just eighteen miles from Nashville, there are plenty of opportunities for big-city cultural events, including a National Football League franchise, the Titans, and a National Hockey League franchise, the Predators. Tennessee levies no income tax other than on investment income and hasn't raised its property tax in fourteen years. A three-bedroom house goes for $270,000, but town houses go for half that.

- *Camden, Maine.* If you like four seasons, this small seaside town will give you plenty of everything. Northern towns such as Camden attract a wide age profile. The presence of a large employer, credit card issuer MBNA, provides job opportunities for all ages and a rich tax base that helps keep local property taxes from soaring. Some other attractive four-season favorites include Boise, Idaho; Petoskey, Michigan; Cape May, New Jersey; Lancaster, Pennsylvania; Door County, Wisconsin; and Sequim, Washington.

Sexual orientation. For gays and lesbians, there's always San Francisco, yet many in the gay community are shut out of that city's comfortable tolerance for alternative lifestyles because of the expense. A typical house runs $700,000, more than twice the price of homes in most parts of the United States. Anyone looking to quit work will have a hard time making ends meet there—even if they keep a part-time job. But with a steady increase of openly gay boomers reaching their power years and looking for the right place to call home, the options are increasing. A dozen or so developers are now planning gay retirement villages from Boston to Santa Fe. New York, Chicago, and Miami are also gay-friendly U.S. destinations, and Toronto, Vancouver, and Montreal are gay-friendly cities north of the border.

For those seeking a somewhat traditional fun-in-the-sun postcareer life surrounded by gays and lesbians there is the Palms of Manasota near Sarasota, Florida (see www.palmsof manasota.com). There's also the Resort on Carefree Boulevard in Fort Myers, Florida, marketed primarily to lesbians. A newer alternative lifestyle development, Carefree Cove in Boone, North Carolina, started selling lots in 2003.

Other gay retirement communities are urban-based, including the planned Stonewall Communities in Boston and Our Town developments in California. And to open the doors to gay retirement in San Francisco for those without a lot of money there is Openhouse, which is developing "a residential community that will welcome all seniors, and honors lesbian, gay, bisexual, and transgender seniors." Openhouse "will be a multicultural hub" with activities that include studying subjects from architecture to finance. In searching for the right gay community, these Web sites are most useful: www.openhouse-sf .org, www.ourtownvillages.com, and www.gaylesbianretiring .org.

My Old School

In a lot of cases you'll find that college towns offer just the right mix of opportunity and cheap living. Dan has a special place in his heart for Bloomington, Indiana:

In my journalism career I have moved more often than I care to remember. One blessing, though, was my stop at the *Bloomington Herald-Telephone* (later renamed the *Herald-Times*) in Bloomington, Indiana, home to Indiana University and once upon a time the fabled basketball coach Bob Knight. I have fond memories of that idyllic hamlet, with its courthouse on a hill at the center of town, where it is ringed with shops, coffee counters, and cafés. Just a short walk east, the university's sprawling campus begins. It was near the town square that I met my wife of twenty years, reason enough for the place to hold special significance. Yet when I examine all the things that made Bloomington so memorable, I find there was more.

Because the university known as IU so dominates the area, a college feel permeates all aspects of life in Bloomington, from coffee-bar chats on current issues to community bulletin boards proclaiming furniture for sale and roommate wanted. "Townies," as the nonstudent population is known, have easy access to lectures, concerts, and continuing education. Housing is cheap. A typical home sells for under $200,000. There are two recreational lakes. Big-time sporting events occur at IU (in the Big Ten conference) and in Indianapolis, which is just an hour to the north. Basketball is religion (the movie *Hoosiers* depicts an authentic Indiana state high school tournament); so is cycling (the movie *Breaking Away* was based on the town's annual "Little 500"). I have often thought of returning to Bloomington in my power years as a base for freelance writing or to seek a faculty position at IU's highly regarded journalism school. All those fond memories—and IU isn't even where I went to college.

Bloomington is unusual in many ways, but the features that make it special—culture, vibrant town square, small-town setting, a young and diverse population—can be found in hundreds of college towns across the globe. So alluring are these features that retiring to your alma mater or some other university setting has become a blistering trend.

As we reach our next life stage many of us will recall those exciting college days and seek to re-create the best parts. We believe that many universities, finding themselves in such a sweet spot, will make the most of it. They have quite accidentally acquired a valuable lifestyle brand and will see aging boomers as an important constituency, offering us not just continuing education and class auditing but also special housing that woos us back to campus. Universities in beautiful small-town settings will seize on the opportunity to get into the lifelong learning business, fashioning special programs and cultural events with specific boomer appeal. Instead of organizing your life around the third tee, you might prefer to do it around a coffee house or lecture hall.

In recent years, dozens of housing communities have sprouted near college campuses to house the growing number of adults who are living longer and looking for a place that will continue to stimulate their minds and bodies. John and Betty Jean Rife found their ideal power years home in Oak Hammock, an adult community with ties to his alma mater, the University of Florida. The community in Gainesville, Florida, offers campus privileges similar to those of faculty, a fitness center, a massage therapy, and a computer lab. John coveted the chance to hone his computer skills, and his wife looked forward to learning how to paint. "We looked at retirement places pretty much all over the South," said John. This one kept the Rifes close to their children as well as to former classmates.

After more than twenty years of living in Southern California, Elliot and Patricia Mininberg thought they would make Santa Fe, New Mexico, their power years home. But when they visited friends who had moved to Charlottesville, Virginia, a college town in the foothills of the Blue Ridge Mountains, everything changed. "We fell in love with the place. It's very peaceful and beautiful, and there are plenty of cultural activities," said Elliot, a professor at California State University, Northridge. They bought a house on the spot even though Elliot returns to California to teach one semester a year. Patricia loves the historic downtown pedestrian mall. Elliot enjoys playing tennis at the Boar's Head Sports Club, which is owned by the University of Virginia but offers memberships to the public. "Everything here—from home and car insurance to utilities and state income taxes—costs about half what we paid in California," says Elliot. Another big selling point is its mild, four-season climate. "In California, one becomes used to day after day of sameness," says Elliot. "Here, the seasons change and the leaves disappear. There's an annual rejuvenation."

When considering any college town, look for one where the town isn't so large that the general population overwhelms and dilutes the influence of the university. The campus should be walking or at least biking distance from the town square. Inquire at the university if events it sponsors are marketed to the general population. Does the school invite the community to participate through reduced tuition for adults for noncredit classes? If you live on or near campus, will you be too close to frat row and unwanted beer bashes? If you live far from campus, will you have convenient transportation, including a place to park?

Here are some of our favorite college towns:

- *Ann Arbor, Michigan.* This is the home of the University of Michigan. Yes, it's cold in the winter, but this midwestern enclave makes up for it in charm. The university is at the center of the town's cultural life, from plays at the Mendelssohn Theater to live music at the Ark. This is another Big Ten school, and its home football and basketball games are marquee events. Yet you are just an hour from Detroit for a taste of big-city life, and an abundance of lakes and beaches are in easy reach. Ann Arbor has 147 parks, a Bicycle Touring Society, and a Ski Club open to all.

- *Eugene, Oregon.* This is home to the University of Oregon, where mature adults can audit classes and attend campus events for one low annual fee. Homes are reasonably priced, and the views in the Willamette Valley can't be beat, framed by the Cascade and Coast mountain ranges and just two hours from Portland and an hour from the Pacific Ocean. "The surrounding area is a nature lovers' paradise the size of Rhode Island and Connecticut combined: natural forests punctuated by volcanic peaks, wilderness inhabited by blacktail deer, elk, redtail hawks, bear, and cougar; and twenty-one state parks, including nine-mile-long Detroit Lake," goes the description in *Money.*

- *South Oxford, Mississippi.* This is home to the University of Mississippi (Ole Miss). William Faulkner and John Grisham have called this home. Oxford is a bastion of southern culture and tradition rife with literary and historical heritage. In addition to the concerts and theatrical performance on campus, nonstudents can attend brown-bag luncheons with visiting notables. There is a local choral group and band, giving musicians an outlet and music lovers easy access to performances.

Living for the City

On October 1, 1947, World War II veteran Theodore Bladykas, along with his wife and fourteen-month-old twin daughters, moved into a brand-new five-room Cape Cod cottage valued at less than $7,000 that had been erected on a sixty-by-one-hundred-foot lot in the middle of a Long Island potato field. All Bladykas wanted was an affordable home away from the increasingly crowded, costly, and crime-plagued city, with room to park a car and flip burgers in the backyard. His simple quest for serenity started a monumental movement. The Bladykases were the first residents of a futuristic, cookie-cutter housing project built on the outskirts of town by the legendary developer William Jaird Levitt, whose Levittown is widely acknowledged as the country's first mass-produced suburb.

As our parents' generation followed Bladykas en masse to the cities' outer reaches, suburban neighborhoods began to dominate contemporary life. Many of our parents were looking for an affordable spot to safely raise a family. With so many men returning from the military, and with nearly four kids per couple, traditional housing in our cities had become scarce, and the Federal Housing Authority and Veterans Administration began offering easy-term loans to those setting up quarters out on the fringes, where there was room to breathe, ride a bike, and throw a football. Later, an expanding freeway system made these homes even more desirable.

Today, the suburbs—once mere bedroom communities—are full of nonresidential activity. Shopping malls, office complexes, and industrial parks blanket both sides of the interstate bypasses that ring our cities, effectively forming thriving suburban downtowns.

Meanwhile, our cities boast vast tracts of defunct industrial complexes, boarded-up storefronts, and underutilized residential neighborhoods. In response, homebuilders have in recent years begun to pick up the pace of reclaiming urban tracts and turning them into desirable neighborhoods for empty nesters looking for some city action. Why not move to the city? Remember, we're going to be able-bodied, relieved of our child-rearing obligations, searching for new adventures, new connections, and—if divorce and widowhood trends continue—maybe even love. The hustle and bustle of city life pack a lot of punch on those fronts. Mass transit means we won't have to drive. Theaters, restaurants, museums, lectures, exhibits, and new friends are only blocks away. If we need to work, we're more apt to find a job we want where there are an abundance of employers. If our dream is to open a small business, the city will supply many potential customers. In the city many of us will rediscover the diversity and action we crave.

Ken, whose career as a public speaker and business consultant has him traveling nearly every week, could live anywhere in the world but chooses the San Francisco Bay Area because he and his family enjoy the diverse and colorful collection of people there. Like many boomers, Ken and his author/speaker wife, Maddy, have begun to consider a second home. But as their children migrate toward college age, lately they've been thinking that instead of the cabin on Lake Tahoe or the condo in Hawaii maybe they'll try a loft in the SoHo district of lower Manhattan or a flat in the Covent Gardens neighborhood of London.

Some of us will opt for our parents' model: an Arizona enclave of same-aged, same-race, same-religion, same-roots folks sharing the same politics and love of tennis and golf. But we believe that for many boomers this sameness will seem like a twilight zone, and a great many of us will seek urban settings for their age and ethnic diversity, the many cultural delights in our cities, and close proximity to social centers such as coffee shops, libraries, churches and synagogues, nightclubs, and restaurants—as well as nearby airports and top-flight medical facilities.

In looking for your ideal urban setting, pay close attention to:

- *Safety.* Find out if crime is on the rise or decline. Pay closest attention to violent crimes. Typically, overall crime rates in a region will track serious offenses. In other words, if the police are taking care of the big crime problems, the little ones tend to take care of themselves. A forceful crime-fighting mayor and police chief can make a big difference.

- *Neighborhoods.* Good neighborhoods are expensive. But they are also the safest as well as a wise investment. Not every place needs to cost a fortune. Look for cities undergoing change. In South Beach, Florida, when a younger, hipper, gay-tolerant class began moving in, the city's old-fashioned conservatives started moving out—creating terrific housing values for those moving in. See if you can spot a neighborhood that can be stepped into at a bargain price.

- *Vibrant city life.* Many of the world's cities have been hollowed out, their once well-groomed neighborhoods of brick flats and town homes transformed into block upon block of affordable housing that gets more affordable every year. In some cities, like St. Louis, planners have tried to make the most of a bad situation, converting vast parts of the city into tourist and recreational attractions, locating professional sports stadiums in the heart of town, and converting a once-bustling train station into a mall. In recent years, the city has shown signs of reviving.

Which urban areas are getting it right? You just can't beat the Big Apple for diversity and culture, and the cleanup begun under Mayor Rudolph Giuliani has persisted. It's refreshing indeed to walk through Times Square newly aglow with neon additions without having to leapfrog panhandlers and prostitutes. Although real-estate prices are high, you can still find relative bargains in Manhattan Valley near Harlem and the East Village in lower Manhattan. If you'd rather have a view of the New York skyline than be a part of it, builder Toll Brothers is putting up several high-rise complexes just across the Hudson River in Hoboken, New Jersey, including the seventeen-story, 326-unit Sky Club. With a twenty-five-thousand-square-foot health club and a French bistro, this may be a next-generation country club.

No city on Earth can top San Diego for weather, and the city is experiencing a mini-renaissance in the formerly desolate downtown area, where beautiful new apartments and condos are being constructed. In the past ten years, this city has been reborn. The newest icon, Petco Park, near the Gaslamp Quarter, opened in 2004. Condos, offices, and hotel towers are rising. The port is now home to four major cruise lines, and the Gaslamp Quarter is a carnival of food, drink, and music. Getting around on foot is easy, and trolley lines link downtown with outlying areas. The Hillcrest neighborhood, north of Balboa Park, is home to a mix of young artists and professionals, and filled with quirky stores and specialty grocers. And don't forget, San Diego has seventy miles of beaches.

Chicago's only claim on weather is that it can be horrible. But when it's nice in the Windy City it's really nice, and the Senior Lifestyle Corporation has been targeting urban retirees there for nearly twenty years at its signature property, the Breakers at Edgewater Beach on Lake Michigan. Atlanta, Georgia, is a clean, warm city with lots of southern charm that has been attracting northerners of all ages in recent years. Three other warm cities that offer a solid taste of urban life and yet have attractively low crime rates and above-average economic growth are Mesa, Arizona; Austin, Texas; and San Antonio, Texas.

Charleston, South Carolina, is frequently mentioned as a great retirement community. It's a mecca of South Atlantic culture and history. There's something for everyone to enjoy in Charleston, be it the unique regional cuisine, the vibrant fine arts scene, the many golf courses, or perhaps the simple and stunning beauty of its miles of beaches. The architecture is truly something to behold, from stately mansions of colonial times to lavish plantation estates. Yet with a population of 101,024 you'll get a taste of the city as well. Charleston offers a lifetime of museums and points of interest to explore, including the Charleston Museum and Fort Sumter.

Not unlike Charleston in size, Providence, Rhode Island (population, 180,000) offers a taste of urban living in a cooler climate with a different set of historical sites—many from the Revolutionary War as opposed to Charleston's Civil War ancestry. Providence is being reborn, with local leaders literally reshaping and energizing downtown with an arts district and new housing. Providence is just forty-one miles from Boston, another attractive urban area that has been pulling folks of all ages back into the city's financial district, Beacon Hill, the Back Bay, and the South End for years.

Outside the States, Montreal, in Québec, Canada, has a great deal to offer. It is about as far south in that country as possible, which means the weather isn't any colder than in the northern regions of the United States. This city offers a delightful mix of French- and English-speaking establishments and is an outdoorsman's dream, surrounded by ski slopes and trails that serve snowmobiles in winter and cyclists in the summer, and lakes that provide year-round recreation. Berlin, Germany, is a cultural mecca and has a massive need for English-language speakers, particularly as teachers. Or consider Cairo, Egypt, where there are many new metro stations and lines being added to an already extensive, surprisingly modern rail system and an extremely low crime rate.

The Modern Nomadic Lifestyle

A generation that came of age with Jerry Garcia's "Truckin'" and watching Peter Fonda and Dennis Hopper chop down the highway in *Easy Rider* no doubt will turn out a decent share of highly mobile retirees. We imagine that 10 percent to 15 percent of us will want to live our power years roaming from city to city, state to state, even country to country, constantly seeking and finding experiences that keep us turned on and young of mind.

Rich people already do it. They have the house in the Hamptons, the pied-à-terre in Paris, and the vineyard in Sonoma or Tuscany, all of which make for wonderful places to stay while they aren't vacationing in Palm Beach or the Caribbean. Of course, the average person can't afford such a lavish lifestyle, but the idea of not being tied down, of continual variety, is certainly a multiplying trend. Many of us will want to fashion some version of this lifestyle for ourselves—and we will have remarkable success in doing so, should we still be working, in part because the Internet will allow many of us to telecommute from anywhere in the world. And since most of us have built a good deal of equity in or have managed to buy the house we live in (the home ownership rate in the United States is a record 69 percent), this asset will give us more financial flexibility than we might have imagined.

For instance, maybe we'll trade in our house in the suburbs (which may have doubled in value since we bought it in the 1990s and tripled or more if we bought in the 1970s) for a condo on a retrofitted cruise ship that constantly tours the globe. We can meet up with it wherever and whenever we choose. Cruise Ship Condos LLC (www.residensea.com) has a floating condo complex with 350 staterooms and all of the usual cruise ship amenities. You can choose a three-thousand-square-foot apartment, an ocean view suite with a balcony, an ocean view stateroom with or without a balcony, or an inside minimum-cost stateroom. An average outside ocean view cabin will cost $70,000 to $100,000. You are free to sublet, or if you prefer, take just a 75 percent, 50 percent, 25 percent, 4 percent, or 2 percent share and have the condo for a commensurate number of weeks each year, like a time-share. The ship travels fifty weeks a year and docks in fantastic places such as Greece, Egypt, Monaco, Spain, France, and Italy.

On board *The World* cruise ship are all the amenities you'd expect. Sports facilities include a complete golf center offering an open-air full-shot driving range and three putting greens, as well as a full-size tennis court—the first on a large ship. Two swimming pools provide a choice of locations for sunning and swimming, and a retractable marina for water sports enthusiasts is at the stern of the ship. The renowned Swiss spa Clinique La Prairie, runs health and beauty clinics, and the ship's seven-thousand-square-foot spa offers complete workout facilities as well as personal trainers and aerobics and dance classes. A variety of restaurants on board serve contemporary French fusion and Mediterranean cuisine as well as seafood, steak, and sushi. Other on-board eateries include a gourmet market and deli and a street café. Chefs are available to prepare meals in residence kitchens. *The World* features rotating exhibitions of fine art and offers seminars on history, geography, oceanography, astronomy, and art. Wherever *The World* sails, residents and guests get an in-depth preview of the local culture, and they have time to explore the destinations, visiting museums or golfing legendary courses.

If living on the open seas is not your thing, consider a time-share, a concept that went mainstream in the 1970s but has not always been seen in a positive light. At the start, revelations of high-pressure sales tactics for shoddy properties hurt the industry's reputation. Difficulty selling shares after an owner had tired of a location, even with solid properties, didn't help. But the time-share market is becoming more credible, efficient, and attractive all the time. Nearly seven million people—62 percent of whom are over fifty—currently own a time-share. Worldwide sales have doubled in the past decade. In our power years, time-shares will provide an easy way to set up a modern nomadic

lifestyle. To get started visit www.find-timeshares.com or www
.timeshares.com

Charles Lampach, fifty-five, lives and works in New York
City but owns seven time-share weeks around the world, including in South Africa, Mexico, Florida, and Massachusetts. "You
know your fixed costs, and it's cheaper than getting a one-week
rental at a comparable resort," he says. Lampach uses his time-
shares purely for vacation right now. But because there is an
active secondary market where he can buy and sell time-shares
(www.tug2.net) as well as an active swap market (www
.intervalworld.com, www.rci.com) where he can trade locations
with other time-share owners, he can envision using his time-
shares as a base to string together months at a time to live, say, in
Mexico this year and the Caribbean next year. "If you have a
good enough week and location it's easy to trade around," he
says. "I'm going to Greece next year."

Time-shares are the closest thing we can get to multiple
houses without spending a great deal of money or becoming
burdened with upkeep. Their premise is simple: for a one-time
cost of a few hundred dollars and an annual fee also of a few
hundred dollars, you own the right to live in a property for a specific week each year. The location and the time of year you purchase are what determine the price. The time-share world is
exploding with activity as people have begun to use them to map
out vacations in interesting parts of the world and, increasingly,
to live on the go for many weeks or months of the year.

For folks with more resources, big-name developers such as
Ritz-Carlton, Marriott International, Hilton Hotels, and Four
Seasons Hotels are marketing vacation clubs, which can cost up
to several hundred thousand dollars to join and charge annual
dues as high as $18,000. But for that price, you get virtually unlim-
ited access to luxury quarters at hot vacation spots around the
globe. A relatively new venture, Exclusive Resorts, offers accom-
modations at thirty of the world's most glamorous locations,

including Big Island, Hawaii; Los Cabos, Mexico; Beaver Creek, Colorado; London; Paris; Tuscany; and the Bahamas. It's not cheap: the one-time membership fee is $375,000 and annual dues run to $30,000 a year. But everything, including groceries, is included for up to sixty days a year, and the typical house you'll stay in has a market value of nearly $3 million.

Maybe time-shares aren't your bag. Try house swapping with someone in the south of France or Hawaii or Southern California or the island of Nantucket or Paris or Brussels or, well, you get the idea. Thanks to the Internet, house swapping is booming, and it definitely has many advantages. For one thing, you can save a bundle by eliminating housing costs from your travel plans. But also appealing is that you will end up living among the real people in real neighborhoods wherever you go because most people don't live in tourist areas—but they may live close to points of interest.

At age sixty, the farthest afield Patricia Snell—a retired secretary living in the United Kingdom—had ever been was a family vacation on the Italian coast. But after the death of her husband, Tom, she decided it was high time to broaden her horizons. Today, thanks to a house swap, she has recently spent a full year in New Zealand. She had initially planned to visit for a month, until she saw an article about a New Zealand family looking to do a one-year house swap. "When I saw that, I thought I had to give it a try. I never dreamed I would be chosen," she says. But within a few weeks she was packing her bags. "After it was all arranged the scale of what I was doing hit me," she says. "I realized it was up to me to go out and make friends and get in among things." She quickly found herself at the center of a new circle of friends. "I had a wonderful time and did a lot of traveling, and after a while I felt like I could have stayed there forever," she says.

House swapping isn't a new concept. There have been home-exchange companies around since the 1950s. But the World Wide

Web has made exchanges easier to access and allows potential home swappers to communicate more effectively through e-mail and to view photos of thousands of properties. "It's not just about saving money," says Helen Bergstein, founder and CEO of Digsville Home Exchange Club (www.digsville.com), which has about four thousand members. "It's the convenience of having a kitchen, laundry, and, in some cases, the use of a car."

House swapping lets you customize your length of stay—one week or one year—as well as amenities to be included in the swap, from a car or boat to privileges at the local swim or country club. You're limited only by your ability to find a willing party on the other side of the swap. And that is getting easier all the time.

Start your search at www.freehomeawayfromhome.com, which has a list of house-swapping sites. Most charge a modest membership fee (under $50), including www.homexchange .com, www.ihen.com, www.holswap.com, and www.4homex.com. You'll need to be flexible to find a fast match. Always exchange a signed, written agreement that spells out just what is included and what isn't (car, boat, computer, wine collection, heirloom china). Who will pay for utilities? What about smoking? Pets? There are a lot of potential issues, and if you're going to worry too much about a stranger in your house, this won't work. On the other hand, it may be nice to have someone watching things while you're away.

There's no reason to remain permanently tied to the home where you reared your children—if you're ready for a change. This can be an ideal time to pull up roots and re-pot yourself to live in a place or in a style you have only dreamed of—and if it doesn't work out, you can move again, changing your address to match your evolving interests and appetites.

The excitement of discovering your new power years residence can begin right now. As you plan vacations, think of getaways as scouting expeditions. Try out a spot with an eye for whether it might suit your power years needs. Look at real estate, medical facilities, recreation, clubs, libraries, and cultural activities that can include anything from museums and concerts to block parties, barbecues, chili cook-offs, and square dances. Don't shy away from snowy regions. You won't be as brittle as your parents and can stand a little inclement weather.

Don't stop at the border, either.

In Belize, a speck of a country next to Guatemala and south of Mexico, the coastline is two hundred miles long, and many areas are sparsely populated, so you can still find affordable beachfront real estate. The people are friendly and the snorkeling is unparalleled. Costa Rica offers a laid-back lifestyle at a reasonable cost and boasts an impressive national parks system. Mexico is convenient to the States and in places such as Guadalajara, Ajijic's Lake Chapala, and the arts community of San Miguel de Allende, large populations of English-speaking retirees are setting up power-years homes.

If affordability is not your top concern, you can't beat France, Germany, Italy, and Spain for culture—and any one of them can serve as a launching pad to explore all of culturally rich Europe. If the English language is important to you, Canada, England, Australia, Ireland, and New Zealand deserve a look. Check out the Bahamas, the Cayman Islands, and the U. S. Virgin Islands for a tropical lifestyle. And if you're a bit more adventuresome, Thailand is an increasingly popular country for retirees seeking a bit of exotica.

7

Achieving Financial Freedom

Money can't buy happiness. But it does buy opportunity and guarantee choice. How well we save and invest today make the difference tomorrow between having to work and choosing to work; between applying for a job as a night watchman and living out our dreams. If an inexpensive lifestyle—or continuing to work until your final hours—is truly what drives you, then you may not need to save much at all. On the other hand, quitting work for good in your late fifties requires a bundle. So it's important to think now about your life goals and how much you'll need to fund them.

Just seventy years ago, when life expectancy at birth was sixty-three years, we didn't need a lot of savings. Social Security and company pensions were sound, and it wasn't a big deal to put away enough savings to supplement retirement programs and live financially secure for the few years we had left after quitting work. But today's life expectancies reach well beyond the seventies. Most of us will see eighty, many will reach ninety, and millions of us are expected to live past one hundred. This is unprecedented longevity, and it changes the financial preparation equation in a big way.

How much more savings will our longer lives require? Naturally, it all depends on how we expect to live. What do we want to do with our later years? Where will we live? How long will we work? To illustrate the impact of greater longevity, we asked mutuals fund firm T. Rowe Price, a leader in clearheaded retirement planning, to work up some examples based on the old model of quitting work for good at age sixty-five. What we found didn't really startle us. But it's instructive to note the degree to which living longer requires additional savings.

In its workup, T. Rowe Price assumed that all savings were parked in a tax-favored account such as a 401(k) plan, broadly diversified among stocks and bonds, and that inflation would average 3 percent a year. They further assumed average historical rates of return, annual pay of $40,000 plus raises equal to inflation, and that in our power years we'll need 70 percent of our final year's income. Conclusion: you would need total savings of just over $200,000 to retire at sixty-five and have enough money to support yourself for five years. But you'd need more than $900,000 for the money to last twenty-five years—a fourfold increase over what your grandparents expected to need.

That's a lot to sock away, and it helps us make two points. Working longer, as we think many will want to, and starting to save sooner are the surest and easiest ways to relieve long-term financial strain and fund your power years dreams.

How to Fund Your New Dreams

Thankfully, there are many new models of retirement emerging to fit your financial profile and the lifestyle you choose. In the years ahead, you'll enjoy boundless ability to customize your mix of work and play and gather the resources you'll need to fund the power-years lifestyle of your dreams. For most, this dream starts with leaving your high-pressure primary career, probably in your early sixties, taking a little time off for fun and reflection, and then going beyond this turning point to launch a whole new chapter in your life.

Choosing to permanently stop working in your early sixties would put the most stress on your bank account. It requires the most savings, and aspiring to this model creates pressure and worry early in life as you try to balance time with family and the hard work needed to save a massive nest egg that will let you go on a rest-of-your-life vacation. An amazing thing happens, though, when you stop thinking of retirement as a permanent nonearning vacation. The moment you commit to continued employment in any form, funding your later years becomes much less stressful. And remember that working at something you enjoy and on your own terms can lead to a later life filled with connections, new relationships, a sense of relevance, and many other rewards.

For true financial freedom, you'll want the resources to do what you want, how you want, and when you want. Key issues will include living and working on your own terms, shifting the balance between work and leisure to stay challenged and keep the cash flowing—but with a lot more time for play, and achieving a state where you become worry-free knowing that you have the capacity to handle the costs of whatever surprises life might throw your way.

Even if you haven't sorted out what will rock your boat twenty or thirty years from now—and most haven't—financial freedom will be the key to liberation in your power years. Depending on what mix of work and play you seek and believe you can afford, the funding requirements shift significantly. If, for example, you've always wanted to teach or coach basketball or plan community events but couldn't afford to accept the lower pay such jobs offer, you may decide to downshift and take such a job when you turn sixty or seventy. That instantly frees you from any herculean savings model in which you'll need to have accumulated millions of dollars, such as you may have come across in popular, yet misguided financial publications.

Traditional retirement planning usually assumes a permanent vacation at what amounts to a fairly early point in our long lives. But just look at how that changes with a cyclic lifestyle. According to the Merrill Lynch New Retirement Survey, if you are a typical fifty-year-old with household income of $62,500 and savings of just under $60,000, you'd need to start today and save 20 percent of your income every year to retire comfortably at sixty-two. If you wanted to retire at fifty-eight, you'd need an impossible savings rate of more than 100 percent! Now look at how the financial requirements change when we introduce a blend of work and leisure into our later years. If you're a typical fifty-year-old and plan to leave your primary career at age sixty-four and work part-time until age seventy-five, you'd need to save only 6 to 12 percent of your pay; and if you wished to work full-time until seventy-eight, you'd hardly need to save at all—just 3 to 6 percent annually.

For the vast majority, the new paradigm will be a three-step process reflecting a phased or gradual retirement. Although the idea has been around for a while, this model is now gaining popularity, often out of financial necessity but just as often out of a desire to remain connected to work and share in the various social and intellectual benefits of the workplace. Here's how it works:

1. Downsize or Downshift Your Career

As you approach the traditional retirement age of sixty-five, you may have paid off the mortgage and finished with child-related expenses, including tuition. You will probably have saved a large portion of what you need for financial freedom. So trade in your demanding full-time job for one that is fun or rewarding, though possibly lower-paying, such as teaching high school, refereeing the town basketball league, opening your own pub, consulting in the creation of Web sites, or leading bicycle tours through Bordeaux. Already, nearly half of all people between ages fifty-five and sixty-four who quit their primary careers take some kind of "bridge" job.

2. Let Your Savings Keep Growing

You're now working less, more on your own terms, and chiefly for fulfillment—but also to cover monthly living expenses. Say you had been making $80,000 a year in your primary career and had managed to save or inherit $500,000. You may be able to cover all of your expenses now on a salary of only $40,000 or less. The key is to leave your savings untouched, if possible in a tax-advantaged investment account, to grow for another five to ten years or longer.

3. Stop Working for Good

When you're in your seventies and that nest egg of $500,000 has grown to $701,000 after five years or nearly doubled to $984,000 after ten (at 7 percent annually), you can scale back your work schedule again or quit altogether. If the idea of continuing to work into your seventies holds limited appeal, remember that working at something you truly love and on your own schedule can have an entirely different feel.

Key Smarts and Tools for Your Financial Survival Kit

There are many aspects to a broad, carefully crafted financial strategy. This critical and wide-ranging subject can by itself fill a book. Indeed, wherever books are sold there are thousands of mind-numbing tomes devoted solely to financial planning. In general, these books do a fine job of laying out the tedious details—and often of sending you into a coma. But smart financial planning doesn't have to be complicated and oppressive. In fact, it can be liberating.

Based on decades of study and research and interviews with hundreds of financial planners, in this chapter we offer a simple, effective, and actionable approach to getting your financial house in order. Our generation's low savings rate and profligate spending mean that in the stretch run to maturity we're going to have to make some adjustments. Because so much of our life is oriented around immediate gratification, the idea of a long-term financial plan may even be a bit overwhelming. But as we live longer and the responsibility to fund our power years increasingly falls onto our own shoulders, it's foolish not to have a workable plan of action.

Ken recounts this illustrative story:

The last time I took my son Zak on a week-long rafting trip down the Colorado River through the heart of the Grand Canyon, our group was dropped by helicopter, fitted with life preservers, and put on a large rubber Zodiac raft. I had the feeling that I was beginning one of the most peaceful and joyful vacations I would ever experience with my son, who was ten at the time (I was fifty). With a warm blue sky above and majestic canyon walls rising nearly a mile on either side, Zak and I lay back and relaxed into dreamy, floating sensations as we began our downstream glide. This is about as good as it gets, I thought.

But within minutes the raft began to convulse as it entered the first of dozens of white-water sections in which the raft felt as though it would be tossed into the air and then submerged beneath the raging and near-freezing water. As everyone held on to their safety straps it occurred to me that besides my son, the most important person on that raft was the guide. Only he knew the river, what lay ahead. From his many previous journeys, he knew best how to navigate through the tough spots—which had taken more than a few lives over the years—and keep the trip fun for young and old alike.

In much the same way, as each of us creates a vision for how we'd like to spend our power years, it can be enormously helpful to have some sense of what lies ahead and how to navigate the journey. Will our ride be smooth and easy, or will we encounter rough water—maybe a troubled marriage, parents needing elder care, or a personal health crisis? When we hit the rough spots, will we be caught off guard, or will we be prepared? Allow us to be your guides as we explore the best route down this challenging river. Here are some simple and interconnected actions that can work wonders:

Don't Count Too Much on the Government or Your Employer

Funding your longevity poses vastly different challenges from anything your parents or grandparents confronted. Not only will you live far longer, you also cannot count on the same elaborate safety nets. Pension systems in many developed nations are growing less secure as the age wave rolls around the world. Longer-lived populations put an extraordinary strain on governments' ability to provide the retirement security they once thought possible and indeed promised to their citizens. In many developed nations there simply aren't enough workers to support a massive retiree generation. This is a widely underappreciated problem. In Canada, for example, a recent poll showed that the average worker expects the Canada Pension Plan to provide an annual retirement benefit of $13,200, when in fact the plan will pay just $9,950 on average.

From Chile and the United States to England, Poland, and even liberal Sweden, governments have been backed into a fiscal corner and are experimenting with new pension models to replace the long-promised, underfunded, and increasingly impossible retirement guarantees they've made. These models incorporate what are known as private accounts, which replace government promises with hard assets in your own name that can never be taken away from you. But for private accounts to fully replace government-promised retirement benefits, you'll have to be a master investor; the burden of retirement security is slowly being shifted to individuals. This seismic change in which citizens lose entitlements but have greater ability to invest—leaves us all less financially secure. But given the mathematical difficulty of maintaining state-sponsored pensions in their current form while boomers worldwide reach their later years and start to draw down the resources of the smaller generations behind them, something had to be done.

Consider Social Security in the United States. Sure, the program is running a surplus and will continue to collect more than it pays out until around 2018. But then we turn the corner and retiring boomers will strain the system to the breaking point. In theory, there is a current Social Security surplus that should get us through our retirement years with few problems. But that's really a kind of hoax. The surplus has been spent on other programs. The funds needed to restore the surplus won't magically appear when the money is needed; they will have to be raised through higher taxes; more government borrowing; or, most likely, a cut in future Social Security benefits.

At one time, the pay-as-you-go system made sense. The government used the tax receipts of current workers to fund the benefits of current retirees. Nothing was set aside; nothing was invested. It wasn't necessary. There were plenty of workers paying payroll tax to support every retiree at a high level of benefits. When the U.S. government cut the first Social Security check to Ida May Fuller back in the Depression era, no one knew what a great deal it would turn out to be for her generation. She had paid a total of just $24.75 in Social Security taxes in her working years. She lived to be a hundred and collected a total of $22,889 in lifetime benefits. No one complained that Fuller was getting almost a thousand times more than she paid. In her day, there were almost forty-two workers for each Social Security beneficiary. The payments weren't a problem.

But in the years ahead, there will be too many retirees living far too long for the system to remain solvent. Instead of 42 workers for every beneficiary back in 1940, there are today just 3.4 workers, and by 2050, the worker-to-retiree ratio will be just 2 to 1. The burden on workers at today's benefit levels will simply be untenable. Beginning in 2008, the first boomers will be eligible for early retirement, and the following two decades will see a rapid rise in the cost of delivering Social Security benefits, from about 11 percent of all taxable earnings to more than 17 percent when the final boomers reach normal retirement age in 2031. To convert Social Security and run it like a traditional pension would require $12 trillion, a staggering amount that exceeds America's total economic output for a year. It just won't happen.

Our generation, whose large numbers and hefty tax contributions made the pay-as-you-go system workable for our parents, will become an enormous burden that younger, smaller generations behind us cannot hope to shoulder. Our private pensions are in similar trouble, and the issues that plague them will only compound as we grow older. Our employers never expected former workers to live into their eighties and nineties.

For that and other reasons they failed to set aside enough money to keep their pension plans viable. Old-line industries from steel to rubber to airlines to autos are particularly hard pressed because they have had to shed assets and shrink their business to remain profitable, and are mathematically unable to support legions of former employees. Failing pension plans are now overwhelming the Pension Benefit Guaranty Corporation, which insures pensions up to a point and has been technically insolvent for years. In all likelihood the PBGC will require a taxpayer bailout within five to ten years.

Whatever your political persuasion, we'd all be wise to rely less on the government and our employers when it comes to funding our retirement dreams—and to rely more on our own strategies and plans.

Spend Less

Most of us have a long way to go in our quest for financial freedom. Having spent freely on plasma TVs and SUVs—choosing to live for today—we have managed to accumulate few savings while becoming awash in debt. Boomers have never been big savers to begin with, but during the boom years of the 1990s we basically stopped saving at all, optimistically figuring that the stock market would keep rising 20 percent a year and, in our plans to build a nest egg, do the heavy lifting for us. That didn't work out so well.

While we were counting on the markets to bail us out, our savings rate plunged to less than 1 percent from more than 10 percent two decades ago. We must do better. More than ever, we're on our own financially. Most of us already earn as much as we are able within our chosen lifestyle and priorities. To save more we need to make do with less than we can afford.

We need to cut our expenses. It's not as hard as we might imagine. All of us have a great deal of control over how much we spend. We can choose to eat out or eat in; live in a big house or a smaller house; drive or fly; set the thermostat at sixty-eight or seventy-two degrees; vacation overseas or near home; join a health club or jog outdoors. How we set up our lives determines what our fixed expenses will be, and little changes can truly add up to big money over time.

Try this for simple but compelling math: if when you were in your early twenties you had started to save $5 a day in a 401(k) account, some forty years later you would have amassed a kitty worth $1.7 million. Financial planner and author David Bach describes this phenomenon as "the Latte Factor," a term he uses so often in his seminars that he trademarked it. The Latte Factor springs from Bach's observation that at coffee chains a latte and muffin (which presumably our waistlines can do without) costs about $5. Some people indulge every day, and if they did nothing more than skip the coffee stop they would save $35 a week, $150 a month, or $1,825 a year. A twenty-three-year-old who starts to save that much money and puts it in a 401(k) account with a 50-cents-on-the-dollar company match would, by age sixty-five, accumulate $1.7 million.

Is there anything in your life that you could cut without suffering too much pain? Try bringing your lunch instead of eating out. That will save $5 a day or more. Quit smoking. There's $7 a day. Can you really taste the difference between a $17 bottle of wine and one that sells for $22? If you use half as much detergent in the laundry, your clothes will get just as clean—promise. And when you cook, make enough for two or even three meals. That way you'll be less inclined to order out the next night. Look hard enough and you'll find things you pay for every day that you just don't need. One big killer is restaurant tabs. We know people who almost never cook at home and have almost nothing in the bank.

The little things really do matter. Thanks to the power of compound returns, if we cut our daily expenses by even a small amount we can save a lot of money over time, and this plan works no matter how much we earn. Too often we find that folks with the biggest salaries are the ones in the most trouble because of the easy credit that banks and card companies throw their way. An affluent household earning $500,000 a year and spending above its means can easily wind up worse off than a middle-class household earning just $50,000 a year but saving $100 each month. How much is enough? As a benchmark, 10 percent of household pretax income is a decent start. And more would definitely be better.

Invest in Your Future

In our live-for-today society, many of us tend to satisfy our current appetites and pay little regard to our future needs or to the way we'd like to live and feel a few years down the road. If we gave more thought to the financial requirements of our future, the balance between today and tomorrow would shift, and while we might have a little less spare cash today we'd wind up having a lot more tomorrow.

Every single month or at every single pay period, write a check to your future self. Think of it as a science fiction story in which you're creating a financial time capsule to be opened in twenty years. How can you afford the things you think you need if you're sending a portion of your income to the future? Maybe you can't at first. But you'll quickly adjust. Just as the amount of junk we save in our attic expands to the size of the attic, our bills tend to expand to consume all of our available income. So pay your future self first, and let your bills eat up what's left.

If you're like most people who try this system, within just a few months you'll find that you've adjusted your spending to accommodate the change. Then when you occasionally have something left over you can treat yourself in good conscience.

Pay Off Your Credit Cards

The burden of debt is a lot to overcome as we put our financial houses in order. In January 1970, Americans carried an average of three credit cards per person and owed $127 million on those cards. Today the average American carries between five and ten credit cards and we collectively owe more than $1.6 trillion—a twelve-thousandfold increase. Although credit cards provide many conveniences and useful functions, they are being abused by too many people. With preapproved direct mail solicitations flooding the market—three billion pieces a year—Americans have more credit cards (over one billion) than the rest of the world combined.

Unfortunately, we're on a fast track to becoming a generation of people like George and Maria Rudd, a Miami couple whom Dan wrote about in a cover story for *Time* under the headline "Will We Ever Retire?" The Rudds could not retire. Together they were earning $280,000 a year but had more credit-card debt ($45,000) than savings ($40,000). George, sixty-nine, and Maria, sixty-two, once cashed in a 401(k) account to buy a $58,000 sailboat. "We live dangerously," Maria confessed. "If push comes to shove, I guess we could live on the boat."

After denying themselves almost nothing through their high-earning years, the Rudds' lives today are riddled with anxiety and missed chances. Through the scourge of credit cards, easy use of a 401 (k) account, and home-equity borrowing, they dug themselves a deep hole of debt from which they may never be able to emerge. The Rudds' experience is all too common, and they are a mournful face of retirement that many of us will see in the mirror twenty years from now if we don't make the right choices.

We all have a bit of the Rudds in us, and it's critically important that we shed our debt-financed lifestyle now. Here's what to do:

- Cut up your credit cards, or at least get them out of your purse or wallet. This does two things: it forces you to pay with cash, which is a proven deterrent to whimsical purchases and may just keep you out of the mall altogether; and it keeps you from digging an even deeper hole. You can't climb out while you're busy burying yourself.

- Consolidate credit-card balances in an account that charges a low interest rate. We're not talking about teaser rates, which may last just three to six months before reverting to nosebleed levels of 16 percent or more. Some cards have fixed rates as low as 10 percent or 12 percent. That's where you want your balance, unless you can get an even lower rate by consolidating debts under a line of credit linked to the value of your house. The interest rate on a home-equity line of credit may be as low as the rate on your first mortgage—6 percent or so in recent years.

- Commit 5 percent of your pretax income each month to paying off the balance. A lot of advisers, such as the popular Suze Orman, would say not to save or invest a nickel while carrying a big credit-card balance, and they have a valid point. When you pay down a credit card that charges 18 percent a year in interest you are effectively getting an 18 percent return on that money. We believe it's more important to get into the savings habit as early as possible.

Now Pay Down Your Mortgage

Debt isn't always a bad thing. The home mortgage was popularized at the turn of the twentieth century by Bank of America founder A. P. Giannini and has done more to foster household wealth than mutual funds, certificates of deposit, interest-bearing checking accounts, IRAs, and 401(k)s combined. Residential real estate is an appreciating asset (rising 6.3 percent a year since

1968), and it comes with many perks, including tax-deductible interest and tax-free capital gains of up to $500,000 for a married couple in the United States. It pays to buy a house, but almost everyone goes deep into debt to do so.

Experts have begun to forecast that in the coming decade, real-estate prices will not appreciate at anywhere near their recent pace—maybe not even at their historical rate. Home ownership still makes sense—we are not among the worrywarts who believe housing prices have reached bubble status, and we don't believe that a broad collapse in the market is imminent. Still, housing price gains have exceeded gains in personal income for a decade, and that is not likely to be sustained. This is not a reason to sell your home and rent. Over the long haul, real estate will most likely continue to appreciate, though at a slower pace. And you have to live somewhere.

With the possibility that housing prices may be less likely to keep rising briskly, it's more important than ever to shed your mortgage debt as quickly as is practical. Many of us, though, are going in the other direction. As interest rates fell sharply in recent years we wisely refinanced our homes to lock in lower rates. But rather than socking away the monthly savings, we spent this bounty on vacations, swimming pools, and SUVs. Even worse, as we refinanced we cashed out our home equity and spent it on even more things we may not have really needed. U.S. homeowners cashed out a staggering $333 billion in the three years ending in 2003, reports mortgage giant Freddie Mac. The only three-year period that comes anywhere near that level was $114 billion for the three years before that.

Don't get sucked into thinking that a steep monthly mortgage payment is a necessary part of life. First of all, you don't have to buy the biggest house you can afford. You can choose to keep your mortgage down by buying a smaller house, refraining from spending your equity, and living within your means. Second, debt is debt whether it's been taken on to own real estate or a fur coat.

The more you pay in interest each month, the less you have to save and invest. So after you have a handle on your credit card debt, start accelerating mortgage payments.

The magic of paying more than you owe really is breathtaking. If you make just one additional payment per year on a thirty-year loan you'll own your house in about twenty-two years. Make two extra payments per year—say, in December and June—and you'll own your house in just fifteen years. Another way to accomplish this is by paying more than you owe each month. By adding just 10 percent to your mortgage payment every month you'll also own your house in about twenty-two years. Another route to the same destination is choosing to pay half of your mortgage every two weeks. Because so many people get paid biweekly, many banks have specific programs to make mortgage payments each pay period. By paying half as much roughly twice as often you effectively make one extra monthly payment per year, and will cut eight full years from your thirty-year payment schedule.

One caveat: don't just send the mortgage holder an extra check whenever you like. To make sure any extra payment gets credited to your principal balance and to ensure that you keep making the payments, tell the bank what you're doing and set up an automatic debit account. You'll soon forget that you're paying more than is required, and you'll be on your way to owning your house more quickly. Don't worry if you plan to move in a few years. The extra payments will help build equity that will come in handy when you sell and buy another house.

Be Clear about Your Potential for Inheritance

Few things in life are as gratifying as passing on wealth to loved ones. Our parents for the most part are doing their best to leave something behind, just as we will strive to do for our children. North American boomers stand to inherit more than $25 trillion over the next twenty or so years, but we won't all get an equal share. Most economists predict that 10 percent of us will receive 90 percent of the transferred wealth. Many of us will get nothing at all. Be mindful, too, that our parents are living much longer, and even if we stand to inherit a large amount, we may not get it before our own retirement years are upon us. Moreover, our parents may struggle with unexpected long-term health problems, causing our inheritance to be spent down and possibly even leaving the family with debt.

If you do get an inheritance, consider it a second and possibly last chance at financial security, and guard it wisely. Don't reward your good fortune with the whimsical purchase of a big new boat or pricey vacation. If you must buy something nice for yourself or your family, limit the cost to no more than 10 percent of the inheritance. This is a chance once and for all to wipe out the interest payments on credit cards and auto loans that have been soaking up so much of your monthly income. You may even use the windfall to pay off your mortgage, recognizing that through easy home-equity lines of credit you can quickly tap that source anytime should an emergency arise.

If you're already debt-free, or after you get that way, the inheritance should be safely stashed in a diversified portfolio, where it hopefully will continue to grow. Depending on your age and health, this lump sum or a portion of it may also be used to buy an immediate annuity to lock in income for life. More on that later. If you're lucky and you inherit stocks or mutual funds already inside a tax-favored savings vehicle such as a Roth or traditional IRA, draw those funds down slowly over your lifetime so they can continue to grow tax-free or tax-deferred.

Max Out Your 401(k)

Now that you're spending less, have your credit cards under control, are paying off the mortgage ahead of schedule, and have gotten real about what you'll inherit, it's time to consider how to make the most of the resources you'll be amassing. Most working Americans have access to a tax-favored, employer-sponsored savings plan. In private business these plans are known as a 401(k). For government and educators the plans are known, respectively, as a 457 or 403(b) plan, all named after sections of the tax code. Make the most of these plans by contributing as much as the law allows (the limit depends on your age, income, and company policy) and by having contributions automatically taken from your paycheck. We're big fans of automatic payroll or bank account debits. Why? Once you set up a plan and you're having contributions automatically deducted, you'll begin building wealth without giving the matter another thought.

Automatic contributions to tax-favored plans are the closest thing to an investment no-brainer we've been able to find. However, just 66 percent (and falling) of boomers who are eligible for a 401(k) bother to enroll, and only one in ten makes the maximum allowable contribution. Of boomers in a 401(k) plan, the median balance is $55,000, which sounds like a decent number until we realize that the oldest of our generation are passing sixty, and 401(k)-type accounts may be their chief savings tool. Meanwhile, one in four of us has an outstanding loan against our 401(k), greatly diminishing the plan's value. And more than 6 percent of us pay stiff penalties to take an early withdrawal because, well, we really needed those Manolo Blahnik shoes.

Vanguard's One-Step program for 401(k) savers is an excellent example of the latest thinking in how to prepare for the next stage of life. Through One-Step you are automatically enrolled in the program's low-cost funds, automatically increase your contributions with each pay raise, automatically have your allocation of stocks and bonds shift from aggressive to conservative as you age, and then get access to advisers on how to best withdraw your money after you retire. We are fans of this approach.

The 401(k)s provide a pure form of a time-tested investment strategy known as dollar-cost averaging. By having money taken directly from your check you'll end up investing a set amount at regular intervals every month or every couple of weeks. But dollar-cost averaging is just the start of what makes 401(k)s a bargain. You're also investing pretax money. Say you make $5,000 a month and are saving 10 percent or $500. The bite isn't as bad as you may believe. To save that $500 in a 401(k), your take-home pay would shrink by just $350 for someone in a 30 percent tax bracket because your contribution comes out before taxes are withheld. Yes, you'll pay tax on this money when you begin to withdraw it in your seventies, but typically that's at a lower rate, and only after the deferred taxes have been compounding for decades.

On top of these advantages, in most plans your employer will match some portion of what you invest, which is even more free money. In our example, if your employer match was 50 cents on the dollar, you'd get an extra $175 each month. The bottom line is that while your take-home pay would shrink by just $350, your savings would grow by almost twice that amount: $675 each month.

Employer-sponsored tax-favored savings plans should always be funded to take full advantage of any employer match. If you can save beyond that, the best vehicle is a Roth IRA (adjusted gross income must be below $160,000 for couples and $110,000 for singles). Roths allow you to save after-tax money, which then grows tax-free for life. While there's no employer match, it's a better deal than a 401(k). But if you don't qualify, max out the 401(k) before looking into other options, such as a traditional IRA, where your contributions may not be tax-deductible. If you are self-employed or have any freelance income, it's also a good idea to take advantage of tax-favored savings plans designed just for you. Those include the individual IRA, Keogh, Simplified Employee Pension (SEP), and Simple

IRA, which boast similar tax deferrals but generally allow for higher levels of saving.

Diversify Your Stocks

Even if stocks deliver subpar returns over the next decade, they will remain an excellent way to build long-term savings. In an environment where stocks return at least 7 percent a year (a cautious projection), bonds likely will produce half of that total return. Cash equivalents such as Treasury bills and money market funds will return even less. So we simply cannot afford to give up on the asset class with the most promise, the one that over time has beaten everything else. According to Ibbotson Associates, a firm that has been tracking market returns for decades, the S&P 500, including dividends, has generated average gains of 10.2 percent a year since 1926. In the same period, government bonds have returned an average annual 5.5 percent; 30-day Treasury bills, 3.8 percent.

You should own enough stocks to be exposed to both large and small companies; those that pay dividends and those that do not; some foreign stocks; and steady growers such as food and beverage companies, which tend to outperform during recessions; and companies that tend have their best years when the economy is booming, such as builders and materials companies. In general you'll need a minimum of fifteen to twenty stocks, making certain that in your portfolio at least ten different industries are represented. Instead of stocks, consider Exchange Traded Funds, a relatively new option. ETFs are baskets of stocks—like mutual funds—but are priced continuously and trade on the stock exchange.

Once you're properly diversified, you'll need to rebalance your portfolio every year. Here's how it works: say your target asset mix is 60 percent stocks, 30 percent bonds, and 10 percent cash. When stocks have a good year and bonds lag, the stocks' value will rise, and your portfolio might tilt to 70 percent stocks, 23 percent bonds, and 7 percent cash. By selling enough stocks and redistributing the proceeds to get back in balance—60, 30, 10—you sell what has done best and buy what has lagged. At some point the asset category that has lagged will pick up the pace again and you'll have bought more while it was down.

Rebalancing truly works magic. It keeps your asset allocation where you want it for safety, and it painlessly forces you to buy low and sell high. You should rebalance not just your total asset mix but also the holdings within your stocks and stock funds—that is, keep your target mix of large companies versus small companies, foreign stocks versus domestic stocks, and growth stocks versus value stocks at the preset levels. We recommend rebalancing once a year, and having a first-rate financial adviser can be extremely valuable in crafting and regularly course-correcting your strategy.

Consider Mutual Funds

Since the Massachusetts Investors Trust, the world's first mutual fund, came into being in 1924 amid howls of skepticism, mutual funds have evolved into our primary means of saving and investing. In all, fund companies globally manage more than $14 trillion, and $3 trillion of that is in tax-favored retirement accounts. In the United States alone there are more than eight thousand mutual funds, more than the number of stocks listed on our major stock exchanges.

With mutual funds, you get professional money management and easy diversification at a fairly low cost. Think of a fund as you would an individual security—one that has built-in diversity and a manager on constant surveillance for things that have gotten too expensive or have become unreasonably cheap.

Investing through funds is simple and effective, but it requires some vigilance. As with individual stocks, your funds should provide exposure to both large and small companies, local as well as international. Your funds should include those focused on growth companies as well as those that pay dividends. The simplest way to achieve all of this is through a single fund indexed to the overall market, offered at well-regarded fund companies such as Vanguard and Fidelity. These firms have made retirement saving about as easy as it can be with special programs for procrastinators and others who don't want to think much about their money.

If you're not in a plan such as Vanguard's One-Step, be sure to augment your stock funds with both long- and short-term bond funds, as well as those that give you exposure to overseas markets, including the emerging markets. Your main charge in investing through funds is to make sure you are diversified. But it's also critical that you pay attention to fees. When stock funds were rising 18 percent a year, it didn't matter much if they charged fees equal to 3 percent of assets—you still earned 15 percent on your money. But when average returns are just 7 percent or so those fees could eat up nearly half of your profits.

So try to buy only funds with an expense ratio below 2 percent, even better below 1.5 percent. Index funds' costs should be well under 0.5 percent. The best mutual fund research is available at www.morningstar.com. Basic fund information can be found at www.ici.org. The clear leader in index funds and low-expense fund investing is Vanguard (www.vanguard.com), whose legendary founder, John Bogle, has railed against high mutual fund fees for most of his professional life.

Bonds and Cash for Stability

Peter Lynch once said that "gentlemen who prefer bonds don't know what they're missing." His point was that while bonds and cash are generally safer, stocks are the best way to build wealth over the long haul. But that doesn't mean we should stand completely clear of all other assets. In fact, studies show that a portfolio with 10 percent in bonds performs just as well as an all-stock portfolio over very long periods. Bonds, which are less volatile than stocks, become even more important as we get closer to the years when we'll be withdrawing from our accounts.

The problem with bonds is that to get a great bull market we have to start with high interest rates. Bond prices rise as interest rates fall, and rates have been falling pretty much since the early '80s, when Treasury bond yields peaked at more than 15 percent. With T-bonds now yielding under 5 percent, there's almost no way to duplicate the bull-market returns of the past twenty years, and with interest rates more likely to rise than to fall from here (bond prices fall when rates rise), we think even average returns for the next few years are a long shot at best.

Still, bonds and short-term cash equivalents such as a money market fund are critical components of proper diversification. Different people have different needs. But in general, if you're fifty, most experts would suggest 70 percent stocks, 20 percent bonds, and 10 percent cash. The stocks portion should be higher (as much as 80 percent) if you're under fifty and lower (as little as 60 percent) if you're fifty to sixty-five. The percentage of assets you should have in stocks past age sixty-five depends on your health, but 50 percent as a maximum isn't a bad target. As you adjust your exposure to stocks, make up the difference from the bond portion. The 10 percent cash figure should remain fairly constant, changing only when you perceive unusual opportunity (adding stocks or bonds) or risk (increasing your cash to, say, 20 percent).

This is basic asset allocation and it is critical to keeping your savings out of harm's way. A 2001 study by the Vanguard Group found that 77 percent of a portfolio's returns are determined by changes in asset mix—not individual stock selection. How can the asset mix be so important? Bond prices often rise when stocks fall. In the tumultuous year of 2002, stocks lost an average 22.1 percent while government bonds gained an average 17.8 percent.

Use a 529 Plan to Pay for Education

Named for a section of the tax code, 529 college savings plans are the best way to sock money away for education-related costs. In the United States, the 529 plans are state-sponsored investment programs. The state sets up the plan with a financial services company and you open an account with that firm. You own and control the account. The child for whom the account is set up is the beneficiary. All investment gains accrue free from federal tax and most state tax as long as the funds are used for qualified education expenses, which include tuition, books, room, and board. Contributions generally are after tax, though some states allow tax deductions. You can open an account for your child, grandchild, a friend's child, a relative, even yourself.

With no age or time limit for when the money has to be used, a child can put off college indefinitely, in which case you have the option of rolling the account over to another child in the same family, defined as nephews, nieces, first cousins, and any of their spouses. The funds can be used at any accredited educational institution, whether it is public, private, two-year, or four-year. Even some international schools qualify. With estimates for four years at a public university in fifteen years running at $100,000 (on the low end) and a private university closer to $250,000, little wonder that cash has been piling into these wonderful savings vehicles. Assets in 529 plans hit $51 billion in 2004, up 74 percent from the previous year. For more, check out www.collegesavings.org and www.savingforcollege.com.

Most developed nations offer some kind of preferred savings vehicle for college expenses. In Canada, for example, you can take advantage of tax-deferred Registered Educations Savings Plans (RESPs) and add to your college kitty with the

Canada Education Savings Grant (CESG), where the government matches 20 cents on the dollar up to $400 a year in your RESP.

Get Lifetime Income

Upon scaling back our work schedules or quitting altogether, one of the first things we should look at is taking 25 percent or 30 percent of our savings and purchasing an immediate fixed annuity to lock in an income stream for the rest of our lives. Again, some fund companies have made it easy to turn your 401(k) plan into an annuitylike stream of income. Fidelity's Retirement Income Advantage program uses a sophisticated "monte carlo" analysis to determine odds of running out of money at various withdrawal rates and uses that information to guide you to a realistic plan.

With immediate annuities you buy a guaranteed income stream that will never change and will last a specific number of years or until you die, if set up that way. Immediate annuities are a tiny fraction of the annuity world, accounting for less than 3 percent of sales. But they are a great way to make sure that your fixed living expenses are covered for life. The downside is that when you die—even if it's soon after you buy the annuity—with most policies the money you paid is gone.

Immediate annuities increasingly are seen among some as a partial solution to the problem of eroding government pension benefits. Some financial services firms have begun to address ways that individuals can better fund their longevity. Annuities can play a big role, helping people create a stream of income that will last a lifetime. One firm committed to a leadership role in this area is Allianz, whose corporate strategy is to be "The Best at Next." We are impressed with Allianz's goal of making annuities more flexible and affordable.

Before long we expect that some of the income from

immediate annuities will become tax-free. A sixty-five-year-old man putting $250,000 into an immediate annuity today would collect about $20,000 a year for life. At seventy, the annual income would be about $22,400. For more on this important tool, check out www.immediateannuities.com.

Insure Your Health and Life

In calculating how much you'll need for financial freedom, you must factor in the somewhat unpredictable costs of health care. In the Merrill Lynch New Retirement Survey, the single biggest fear of the boomer generation is not being able to pay for health-care costs—ranking ahead of major illness or going to a nursing home and, incredibly, three times more worrisome than death itself. As we live longer, health-care costs will consume a greater share of our savings than they did for any previous generation.

At the least, we should expect to pay higher premiums, deductibles, and copays. A study by the Employee Benefit Research Institute (EBRI) shows that a fifty-five-year-old retiring today will need $83,000 to cover typical group insurance premiums such as those at work plus out-of-pocket expenses for ten years—just to get to age sixty-five, when Medicare kicks in. The amount needed for ten years of individual coverage if we don't qualify for a group plan is as high as $256,000 for someone with a chronic condition. Once covered by Medicare, you're not off the hook. You'll need to figure out how to pay for drugs and other services that Medicare doesn't cover, and supplemental coverage could run a total of $116,000 for a sixty-five-year-old through age eighty, says EBRI.

If either you or your spouse works, the best deal is through an employer-sponsored plan. You also can get retiree health benefits from your former employer for eighteen months. This extended coverage isn't cheap, averaging $260 a month for an individual and $676 for family coverage. When extended coverage runs out, contact several top carriers such as Blue Cross/Blue Shield or find a local insurance broker who can price policies. A Web site such as www.insure.com offers tips and quotes.

As for life insurance, it's wise to keep things simple. There are two basic types of policies: whole life and term. Both provide a guaranteed payment to dependents upon our death. But whole life, sometimes called universal life, adds a savings feature that gives it a cash value above and beyond your death benefit. You should buy enough insurance to provide financial security for your children until they're on their own, and for your spouse for as long as he or she lives.

As far as Dani Rhoton knew, her husband, Bud, an ex-marine, was in good health. But he died in his sleep at age forty-five. "I was devastated. Totally lost," the mother of four told the *Seattle Times*. Bud hadn't a nickel of life insurance, and his family quickly came to rely on the Salvation Army's Homeless Family Assistance Program. Dani couldn't afford day care while she was at her cashier's job, and when the kids started getting in trouble in school, she recalls, "I couldn't handle it." She quit her job, triggering a downward spiral of unpaid bills and bad credit. Ultimately the bank foreclosed on her mortgage and took the house.

How much life insurance is enough? Make sure that all debts—mortgage included—can be paid off immediately. Also make sure the benefit is big enough to meet any predictable future lump-sum expenses, such as college tuition or your funeral. On top of that, you'll want a big enough chunk of money to generate monthly income to cover all living expenses for your dependents. Figure another 10 percent to 20 percent for future inflation. The final number can be a whopper. To generate just $60,000 of yearly income you'll need a life insurance benefit of about $750,000. And that's just to provide monthly income; you'll need another kitty to pay off the mortgage and other debts.

Take Care of Long-Term Care

The final piece of the savings and insurance puzzle is long-term care, which covers the cost of a stay in a nursing home or extensive in-home services. These costs are not covered in basic health plans and can leave your spouse and/or your children penniless. Medicare and various supplements provide only limited coverage; Medicaid does not kick in until your own resources are all but exhausted. About 30 percent of nursing home expenses are paid out of pocket because so few think to buy this important coverage when they are able.

Surprisingly, 45 percent of those who receive long-term care are under sixty-five, so this isn't an issue to be put off much longer. Indeed, the costs of this insurance rise so rapidly after age fifty-five that it's best to purchase a policy by then. In a typical case, a fifty-five-year-old would today pay $1,500 a year for long-term-care insurance. If this person waits until age sixty to buy the insurance, the yearly premium jumps to $2,560. Consider that in major cities the average cost of a nursing home stay runs $275 a day, or more than $100,000 a year, and a MetLife survey in 2004 showed that nursing home costs were rising 6 percent a year—more than twice the pace of inflation.

Long-term-care insurance can help preserve your independence by protecting the savings and assets you've spent a lifetime accumulating. At a minimum, you should have enough coverage to pay for one full year of nursing home or home health care coverage, including intermediate and custodial care. But more is better. The average length of a nursing home stay is 2.4 years.

Have the Right Directives and Documents in Order

More than 50 percent of older adults die without a will. This is senseless. There are three basic documents we all should have to

ensure that our intentions are honored after we become incapacitated or pass away: a will, a living will, and a power of attorney.
The most important is a will. We should have had a lawyer draw
up the first one years ago, when we had our first child—if only to
name who would get custody should we die prematurely. But we
were young and felt immortal, and many of us never got around
to it. Well, no more excuses. There's no telling how a state court
will divide our assets if we don't leave instructions. For example,
your kids may immediately get half of everything even though
your spouse survives you. That may not be the way you would
want it. A proper will keeps your estate out of the wrong hands
and ensures that it will be put to the uses you desire.

Fred, a firefighter in Syracuse, New York, died in the line of
duty in 1996 and would have been sorely disappointed at the
legal tussle that followed his death. He left behind $89,000—but
not a will. Fred had had a bank teller scribble on his savings
account documents that if anything were to happen to him his
money should go to his brother, whom he trusted to pay for his
daughter's education. But without a proper will, Fred's ex-wife
and her new husband, who had adopted Fred's daughter, staked
a claim. Ultimately the daughter was seen as the rightful heir—
but not before a long fight, and even then there were no controls
put on how she could spend the money.

A will is especially important in gay and lesbian unions,
which many states do not recognize for estate purposes. A life
partner may be left with nothing. But even in traditional families
many problems can occur when there is no will. In-laws may end
up with the same rights as your flesh and blood; your small business could end up in the hands of partners who hate each other;
and the government could end up collecting a lot more tax than
necessary. Certainly, if you have any special considerations, such
as a dear friend or longtime coworker, they'll get nothing without a will.

You'll also want a living will or health-care power of attorney.

A living will spells out exactly what medical measures you approve to keep you alive should you become incapacitated; a health-care power of attorney empowers a loved one to make such decisions on your behalf. The heart-wrenching Terri Schiavo case in 2005 drove that point home—she had no such written documents, leading to a nasty fight between her husband and her blood relatives. Finally, you should have a durable power of attorney, which authorizes a loved one to make financial decisions on your behalf should you become unable. These documents should be prepared by a lawyer who specializes in family legal matters. It's becoming increasingly simple and appropriate, though, to prepare basic legal documents on your own using software such as Quicken's WillMaker Plus, Kiplinger's WillPower, LegalZoom, Family Lawyer, or BuildaWill. For a free sample of how these documents should be written and what they should include, check out www.easylegalforms.com.

Seek Professional Help

The good news is that the financial services industry has heard the wake-up call and is attempting to shift its style and purpose away from sales to solutions. Helping you plan and envision your dream retirement is the key new ingredient. In a nicely done commercial from American Express Financial Advisers (now called Ameriprise), investors are asked to describe their ideal financial adviser. Their response: guide, teacher, confidant, mentor, ally, motivator, and coach. Of course, while we surely don't expect this industry to lose its profit motive, it is coming to realize that unless it helps members of our generation fund our individual retirement dreams, however straightforward or irregular they may be, financial firms will be missing a massive opportunity.

A lot of us think we can make financial planning a grand do-it-yourself project, and 70 percent of boomers do not currently have a financial advisor. But survey after survey shows that folks who have spoken with a financial adviser are more prepared financially for their later years, and that those who are prepared are 2½ times happier, more optimistic, and half as fearful, and they even expect to live longer.

The Next Steps

Take a deep breath. Sure, you have many challenges. Our private pensions are flirting with insolvency, and blue-chip companies from Morgan Stanley to United Airlines to U.S. Steel are scaling back benefits. Government entitlements worldwide are heading for trouble. Stocks, bonds, and real estate might produce lackluster returns in coming years.

Still, we're an inventive and prosperous generation, and through tax-favored, sponsored savings programs and college plans you have ample opportunity to reach financial freedom. Your biggest problem is getting started and sticking with it. Many folks who don't command big salaries feel like they don't have the means to put anything away; they give up without a try. Others make big bucks and feel that they needn't bother.

Both are wrong. The key is having a vision, forming a plan, and committing to do what it takes to make your power-years dreams come true. In most cases, starting slow with the techniques we've described is all that's required.

But you must get started now. The big secret is that you don't have to make a lot of money to build a suitable nest egg. You just have to think about your dream version of retirement and what you'll need to fund it. Start today with a regular investment program and a renewed determination to avoid excessive debt. The future is yours.

8

Leaving a Legacy

A few years ago *Time* magazine put the name Bill Gates on its list of the world's one hundred most influential people. Surprising? Hardly. Gates is the cofounder and chairman of mighty Microsoft, and the world's wealthiest individual with a net worth of nearly $50 billion. Yet in this case, Gates was not being singled out for his position atop the world's dominant software company, nor did his selection have anything to do with his unparalleled personal assets. Gates, a square-in-the-middle member of the presumably self-centered boomer generation, was chosen for his enormous generosity. He has given billions of dollars to charities around the world, with the broad goal of improving the health and education of the less privileged.

Think of Gates as sounding the charge for our generation. He is making the world a better place with his money, yet that doesn't seem to be quite enough for him. He's also spending many hours thoroughly researching the causes he chooses to fund. As legendary investor Warren Buffett comments: "Bill has become a walking encyclopedia of medical knowledge. He reads many thousands of pages annually so that he can learn how to attack the world's most dangerous illnesses. . . . Melinda [Gates], for her part, travels the world so that she can understand what a check from Seattle is actually accomplishing ten thousand miles away."

Money, yes—in spades. But time, thoughtfulness, knowledge, and passion are things you will have in abundance as you'll have the incredible opportunity to leave the workaholic world behind and reflect on your life experiences and how you can best put them to work. Intel cofounder Gordon Moore has given over $7 billion to education and the environment. Money manager George Soros has given nearly $5 billion to promote his vision of free societies around the globe. Ted Turner, Michael Dell, and mutual fund entrepreneur James Stowers have each given more than $1 billion to their favorite causes. Most folks can't make that kind of financial impact, but you can still make a difference, and do so in ways that are both enjoyable and rewarding.

Aha, you may say. Mind-bending wealth is the key to largesse, as is the case with anyone who gives in large amounts. After all, you must have billions of dollars in order to give away many millions. Right? Well, no. Consider another *Time* honoree: Boston builder Tom White, who made *Time*'s list recognizing folks who were exemplary in various walks of life. In helping to compile the list, Dan had the pleasure of interviewing and later writing about White, who was named America's best philanthropist. White started giving away money almost before he had any. Over five decades he dispensed with more than $50 million.

What makes White so remarkable is that his net worth at the time the story appeared was just $8 million, and on the way to being "given down" to less than $3 million. White, over his life, had given away 94 percent of his potential net worth. He only stopped giving, he said, so he would not threaten to become a burden to his children in later years. "People overemphasize what I'm doing," the reclusive White said when told he was being honored. "I get tremendous pleasure out of giving."

So, it seems, do a lot of us—and not just giving money but also things that may be even more valuable: time, skills, compassion, knowledge, values, and wisdom. Ken once asked President Carter what motivated him to give so much back to the world. Carter spoke to Ken of the "blessing of giving"—he said the harder he and Mrs. Carter work at giving, the more they feel blessed by the results. Giving of themselves, he said, made them stronger. "Every time we thought we were making a sacrifice for others, it has turned out to be one of our greatest blessings," Carter said. "In other words, we have gotten more out of it than we have put into it. You just try it, even if it's nothing more than going to a public hospital and rocking a baby for two hours a week. It's an expansion of life, an encounter with new people who are potentially friends. And so it's a learning process, an exciting process that gives you new and expanding life experiences."

Jimmy and Rosalynn Carter are not alone. In every town, in every apartment building, church, gym, and community center, you can find role models who are giving back to their families, communities, and to society at large. New generations of high-spirited, motivated men and women who, with their deeds and actions, are clearing a new and more hopeful path to our future. To us, these are the real exemplars of what the power years might be.

We believe that once tens of millions of us become unshackled from the rigors of careers and child rearing, our basic desire to be involved and contributing will manifest in all manner of volunteerism. According to a time-diary study conducted by the University of Maryland, retirement frees twenty-five hours a week for men and eighteen hours a week for women. How much golf or pinochle can you play?

Our generation has so many talents, and we have become so accustomed to the satisfaction of putting those talents to work that the notion of helping others can build into a tidal wave—a revolution. Each of us will have the opportunity to help turn our generation's legendary self-indulgence into something useful as we discover the psychological, social, even spiritual rewards of giving back. Like Bill Gates and Ted Turner and many others who are well off, if would be great if you gave money to causes that matter to you. But that's not the only way to make a contribution.

It's been our experience that those who give something back feel best about themselves while those who focus on how much they can take are never quite satisfied. Takers keep looking for more; givers are nourished by their good acts. Sadly, those who take more than they give often fail to recognize their own self-ishness. Sometimes each of us needs to look in the mirror and see what's true about ourselves. Have we become too self-centered? Are we giving enough? Can we reset our taking/giving equation to match the extra free time we'll have in our power years?

In the years ahead, you will have the opportunity to sort through the next chapters in your life and make important deci-sions about your existential priorities. Ultimately, we believe, the purpose of a longer life may not only be to remain young longer—it may also be to have more time to give back.

How much, why, and where you give are your own business. You may want to give money until it hurts. You may want to be personally involved and give so much of your time that you don't get enough sleep. You may be motivated by taxes or estate planning or by an inner voice or by an experience in your own life or a need you've personally witnessed. Pressed for an expla-nation on his philanthropic exploits, White admitted that one of the things that drove him to give away his fortune was that once he became rich, he started hanging around with rich people and he didn't like them. By giving his money to charities even as he was making it, he avoided being part of a class that did not suit him. That's an unusual motive, certainly. And in fairness to White, avoiding being really rich was just a small part of what drove him. As a young man with just over $1,000 to his name, he once gave away $700 to the needy on Christmas Eve. Giving is in his DNA.

Giving is in your DNA, too. You just have to discover what kind of giving moves you most and then work those too-long-dormant muscles. Ours is the most schooled generation in history, and we have lived during unparalleled prosperity and largely unfettered global travel. The world has shaped itself around our bulging numbers, expanding longevity, and increasing wealth. You have acquired wisdom, valuable skills, and keen insights along the way—all of which can be shared and passed on as you give something back in ways that will be both beneficial to your community and meaningful to you.

In addition to money, you can give:

Time. Jean Jones found new meaning in her life by volunteering to be a foster grandparent to second and third graders at McPhee Elementary School in Lincoln, Nebraska. Now, instead of sitting in her apartment and worrying, she stays busy helping youngsters with math problems, reading, and spelling. "I tell everybody I've never had such a rich, rewarding job as I have now," says the woman known throughout the school as Grandma Jean. "You get so much back. This job gets me up in the morning and gets me going. It's great."

Nicholas is one of Grandma Jean's foster grandchildren, and he regards his time with her as the highlight of his day. With busy parents, Nicholas doesn't get the supervised reading at home that he'd like. "This is like having another grandma," he says. "It's a lot funner to be reading with somebody." Jean can read the appreciation in Nicholas's eyes, and it's all the payback she'd ever ask. But she gets more. "First thing in the morning, even the little boys come up and hug me," she says, beaming.

Doris recently flew to Belize to assist the Oceanic Society in a research project on porpoises. "We had chores, like writing down behavior, taking depth readings, and using global positioning devices," she says. "But there was plenty of time off to snorkel, too." Even though she is a volunteer and had to pay her way (many of her expenses were tax-deductible), Doris plans to keep volunteering like this. "I've been to Borneo tracking orangutans, and I want to see the lemurs in Madagascar before they're extinct," she says. "There's an awe about creation you can't find in a museum, and the satisfaction that comes from doing something helpful can't be measured."

Skills. Noreene James of Wasilla, Alaska, always wanted to be a nurse and loves to take care of people. She believes that allowing those who are ill to remain in their homes increases their longevity and quality of life. Through the Experience Works program she is able to get the continual training she needs to keep her nursing assistant license as she works toward becoming a registered nurse. Meanwhile, she revels in being able to provide at-home assistance for five clients whom she helps with daily activities including grocery shopping and exercise. Betty, from Phoenix, Arizona, enjoys a different calling. A lifetime educator, she has always wanted to make a difference in the lives of children. Today she is a dean of students emeritus at a local school. She stays current through courses at Phoenix College and Arizona State, and focuses on fund-raising for scholarships for inner-city children. She visits at-risk students in their homes to talk them out of dropping out of school.

Doug Robinson, sixty-one, is a lawyer living in Washington D.C. He has enjoyed a long and fruitful career as a litigator with the powerhouse law firm Skadden, Arps, Slate, Meagher, & Flom. About ten years ago, Robinson began to feel it was time to start giving something back. Throughout his career he had found small amounts of time to take on pro bono cases, defending those who could not afford a lawyer. He longed to devote more time in that area. "I wanted to focus on doing things that would be a public service," Robinson says, adding that he'd felt he'd already accomplished just about everything he'd set out to accomplish in his field. Besides, he says, "I came to find that my pro bono work was the most fascinating work I was doing."

So he cut a deal with his firm allowing him to spend 40 percent of his time defending the indigent. His appetite for this vocation had been whetted in 1988, when he defended a man wrongly convicted of murder in Texas and who was just two days from being put to death. "We not only saved his life, we got him released," says Robinson, who is morally opposed to the death penalty. There was not a single piece of physical evidence linking the man to the murder, and the prosecution's main witnesses were a jailhouse snitch who swore he heard the man confess and an eight-year-old whose story changed many times. "His original defense lawyer was incompetent," Robinson says.

It took five years, and during that time the man twice more came within days of being executed, but in 1993 the man was exonerated and set free. Since then Robinson has focused most of his pro bono work on death-row cases, which he finds both morally rewarding and intellectually challenging. "I felt like I needed to give something back to my community, and I continue to feel that way more and more every day."

Wisdom. After the breakup of a stormy marriage, Ann was seeking something more meaningful than a fun adventure. She wanted to give something back to the world, and she found her calling as a volunteer teacher for the Peace Corps in the impoverished country of Mali in West Africa. She was adopted by a Muslim family, was given a Malian name, and learned to pray in the village mosque. As "professor of English" at the state teachers college in Mali's capital of Bamako, she teaches debate, black

American history, and the philosophy of Emerson and Thoreau to French-speaking African students.

Several years ago, *Fortune* ran a thoughtful story about mature adults and retirement with the provocative title "Candy Striper My Ass." The article was prescient—it indicated that there were probably millions of retirees who would love to contribute their talents and abilities, but that the volunteer industry hadn't yet developed the vision or infrastructure to deploy an army of highly educated, seasoned, capable adults with far different hopes and skills than energetic young beginners. So you need to persevere.

You Are What Survives of You

Unless you find ways to give something back and keep contributing in your later years, you will help cement our generation's reputation as a bunch of narcissists. If you choose to leave a legacy—and we are hopeful that the majority of our generation will—you can help us all be remembered with regard and admiration because you'll be using your power years to make the world a better place.

Carl Jung wrote that mankind cannot reach a state of true fulfillment until late in life. Only after years of growing and continual learning may we finally reach "individuation," which is the state of being all that you can be. Jung proposed that adulthood provided a new stage of discovery, one in which you cultivate aspects of your personality that had been neglected earlier in life, including your propensity to give something back.

The great twentieth-century thinker, psychologist, and philosopher Erik Erikson went even further. He concluded that each successive stage of life involved the letting go of concerns and responsibilities that attended earlier stages. In doing so you are able to assume new challenges, and only after many years of continually developing as a person can you attain true wisdom. For Erikson, the final challenge is to give something back. The most actualized, or fully developed, adults reach the point where their greatest satisfaction in life is giving, Erikson asserted. Erikson felt that this stage of life afforded the special opportunity to complete nature's life cycle by allowing each individual to contribute what he or she has learned back to society. He wrote, "We can look back over a long past, and so doing helps us understand our lives and the world we live in."

Erikson's ideals reflected his mounting concern about the growing potential uselessness of elders in modern society. He felt strongly that the whole society suffers, not just the individual, when mature adults are removed from the tapestry of intergenerational life: "When no challenges are offered, a sense of stagnation may well take over. Others, of course, may welcome this as a promise of respite, but if one should withdraw altogether from generativity, from creativity, from caring for and with others entirely, that would be worse than death."

In earlier centuries, it was common for members of all age groups to live, work, and socialize together. The fragmentation of modern times, however, has eroded the thousands of intergenerational contacts that used to be a natural part of life. By giving of oneself in this fashion, there is the opportunity to reconnect the social fabric and experience the gratification of meeting what Erikson felt was life's final challenge: "I am what survives of me."

As you seek your own version of self-actualization, you will have the opportunity to transform your retirement years from a period of retreat and entitlement into your power years. With extended longevity, a true wealth of life experience, and a reignition of your idealistic engines, we hope you will also find that giving can be its own reward.

Bridging the Generational Divide

Can we really turn the corner on self-indulgence and become, perhaps, the most generous generation in history? It's not so far-fetched. Boomers have long displayed a passion for causes, protesting the status quo since the Vietnam War and civil rights movement. We've railed against injustices and impracticalities for as long as we've been alive. We took on environmental issues, and forced things like cleaner coal-burning facilities on energy companies and seat belts and air bags on automakers. We fought for proper disposal of nuclear waste and we railed against the nuclear arms race. We've questioned every war in the past forty years, challenging our government with an unprecedented level of public scrutiny. We fought for equal pay and opportunity for women and minorities. We even turned our profit-minded commercial enterprises into organizations with a conscience by rewarding them our business when they agreed to restore the Statue of Liberty or support the Special Olympics.

Now, as we approach our power years, we are already far bigger contributors of money and time than you might imagine. Today, middlescent men and women are already paying more than 60 percent of all taxes and are therefore funding support for tens of millions of kids and tens of millions of seniors while paying for our military and nearly everything else. And considering the long hours that most of us are putting in at work, our generation is—surprise—the most generous with the thing that is most dear at this point in our lives: time. Data from the Bureau of Labor Statistics show that boomers are actually logging in more volunteer hours than any other age group. We are most likely to volunteer with kids' after-school programs, for local political causes, and for a wide range of church, civic, or other organizations in our communities.

Disappointingly, volunteer rates are the lowest precisely among those with the most time on their hands: those currently sixty-five and up. While some of today's mature adults are living productive and useful lives, far too many are not. Today's average retiree watches forty-three hours of television per week, with 80 percent not working. Our long-lived men and women—the world's fastest-growing natural resource—is profoundly underutilized. And while we'd agree that there's something funny about retirees' bumper stickers that proclaim "We're spending our kids' inheritance," there's something shameful about it as well.

Ken asked President Carter if he felt that older adults were giving enough back. "No," Carter said. "But it's not a deliberate attitude of selfishness. It's primarily the timidity that we feel in taking an unpredictable step into a greater life. There's a hesitancy we have about reaching out to someone else in an attitude of friendship. I think that's the main thing—we get too timid to share part of our lives with strangers or with people whom we don't understand and we build an increasingly diminishing cocoon within which we survive."

Today's retirees' lack of social involvement and contribution to younger generations is both unfortunate and unsustainable. Modern society desperately needs to replant the experience, wisdom, and resources of adults into the fields of tomorrow. We need new roles for maturity that not only allow people to be free to reinvent themselves and do their own thing but also ones that encourage them to stay connected and to contribute. And if new generations of young workers are to feel good about giving up a sizable portion of their income in the form of Medicare and Social Security, you can bet they're going to feel better about such sacrifices if they feel that older adults are making some sacrifices, too.

Broadly speaking, despite their considerable wealth and security, most members of our parents' generation have unfortunately adopted a non-Eriksonian mindset of entitlement. We could be heading for an intergenerational train wreck if we don't better balance the giving and taking between the generations.

For example, in the United States, since 1970, total federal spending on Americans over sixty-five has increased from 15 percent of the entire budget to a gargantuan 35 percent (and climbing) today. Elders—whose poverty level has plummeted in recent decades from 30 percent to 10 percent—annually receive $17,700 each from the federal government. How odd that children under eighteen, who suffer with a scary 20 percent poverty level, receive only $2,500 each. And so for every dollar in federal funds that seniors receive, kids get only 14 cents! This doesn't seem fair.

MIT's Lester Thurow agrees that such an imbalance could ultimately have a destructive effect: "All successful societies need to make long-term investments in education, infrastructure, and the basic research that leads to growth industries like biotechnology and new business opportunities on the Internet. How is this going to happen when the largest and most powerful voting bloc is the elderly, who know that they stand no chance of seeing the benefits of these investments?"

Thurow's concerns are real: during the past twenty years, government investments in infrastructure, education, and research and development have fallen from 24 percent to 15 percent of the federal budget. During that same period, government spending on entitlements for the elderly grew by a whopping 253 percent. As our massive generation barrels toward our power years, we have a choice: we can either use our huge size and political clout to drain society of its coffers, or we can use our wisdom, skills, and newfound free time to give something back and by so doing, establish a more equitable balance between the generations.

Needed: A Worldwide Elder Corps

For more than twenty years, Ken has been campaigning for the creation of a Worldwide Elder Corps, which he hopes to participate in when he and his wife become empty nesters and have more free time. He envisions this initiative as something like a Peace Corps for folks in their power years. In his 1989 book *Age Wave*, Ken wrote: "I strongly believe that we should create an organized Elder Corps. . . . At local, state and federal commissions on aging, at legislative hearings, and at the conventions of AARP and other organizations, we hear how much is being done for the older citizen. But at the same time, we need to hear more about what older people can do for young people, for their communities, and for one another."

Nearly every idea that Ken promoted in that somewhat prescient book, from the emergence of a mature-oriented marketplace to the importance of lifelong learning to the challenge of reforming Social Security to the wonders of the new multigenerational family, has become part of the current fabric of everyday life. Yet political leaders remain in large part too frightened to challenge the elderly to a higher purpose and prefer to treat them in a paternalistic and entitlement-oriented fashion. And, with great frustration, we have observed that most media writers, reporters, and producers in this youth-oriented and youth-populated industry can't seem to envision mature adults as having anything to give. They'd much prefer to feature a story about the seventy-five-year-old with new breast implants than a story about her sister who is running a preschool for underprivileged kids. Perhaps, with the steady aging of our society, the time for a new, more enlightened view of the "purpose" of maturity has ripened.

The goal of an Elder Corps would be to place millions of caring and experienced mature adults in settings where they can share their expertise as artists, businesspeople, administrators, managers—you name it. Too many older adults sit idle in their homes while there are tens of millions of young people who are considered at risk without funding or human resources to help them.

Through the work of an Elder Corps, Ken hopes that our

generation will establish a new Eriksonian model for aging in which we more actively pass on our wisdom and talents. We recognize that there are hundreds of local organizations throughout the world that already draw upon the time and resources of mature adults. But many of these terrific programs lack the funding, infrastructure, promotion, and participation needed to flourish. Some of the better known volunteer organizations that we applaud include:

- *Service Corps of Retired Executives.* Known as SCORE (www.score.org), this group is run by the U.S. Small Business Administration and is made up of ten thousand retired executives who provide free business consulting services to struggling small businesses at nearly four hundred chapters across the United States. When he retired, Frank Leibold expected he'd write his first book and spend more time golfing, fishing, and visiting his grandchildren. But Leibold soon found himself wanting to return to the world of work. "I just want to give back my experience," Leibold told *Fast Company*. "I want to help new entrepreneurs and small business owners to become successes." Today Leibold is one of twelve hundred online counselors volunteering for SCORE. From his home in Myrtle Beach, South Carolina, Leibold works with struggling business managers around the world. Leibold enjoys the process of figuring out how to help. He must continually ask for specifics: What is the target market? How will you promote the product? How will you use the Web? Making sure he understands their real needs is a challenge. The reward is helping them get it right.

- *Experience Works.* This group (www.experienceworks.org) traces its roots to 1963, when President John F. Kennedy decided to make poverty a focus of his 1964 reelection campaign. His project Green Thumb, geared at putting displaced farmers back to work by planting and beautifying the nation's highways, became part of President Lyndon B. Johnson's official War on Poverty. Today, Experience Works provides training and employment to low-income adults. The group focuses on teaching and building skills in high-growth occupations such as health care and computers.

- *Generations United* (www.gu.org). A leader in the field of bringing generations together through volunteerism, this nonprofit organization focuses on promoting university and other programs that appeal to all generations. Its goal is to provide a forum for those working with children and older adults to explore areas of common ground while celebrating the richness of each generation. The organization's core belief is that young people can relieve isolation, loneliness, and boredom among isolated adults while they, in turn, can be a positive role model for youngsters.

- *Senior Corps.* This group (www.seniorcorps.org) recruits adults to serve in a variety of missions, such as acting as foster grandparents to read with and counsel at-risk youths and as social companions who spend time with homebound seniors. Volunteers earn a small stipend and are asked to commit to twenty hours per week. Today, 30,000 adults are in the role of foster grandparent to some 275,000 youths, and 15,000 adults visit some 60,000 shut-ins each year.

Many nations are aging ahead of the United States. As you might imagine, power-years volunteerism has begun to take off around the world. The Global Volunteer Network (www.volunteer.org.nz) places volunteers in community projects in Alaska, China, Ecuador, El Salvador, Ghana, India, Nepal, New Zealand, Romania, Russia, South Africa, Thailand, Uganda, and Vietnam. Amizade (www.amizade.org) places volunteers in Brazil and Bolivia for community service for up to three months. Canada World Youth (www.cwy-jcm.org) places Canadians in service projects around the world for stints of up to eight months. There are hundreds of such organizations spanning the globe. For a list go to www.idealist.org or www.transitions abroad.com or www.globalcitizens.org or www.volunteer match.org.

A recent development in efforts to bring the generations together is the shared site, where institutions geared to the young and to the old are brought under one roof to enrich the lives of both generations and foster a better understanding between them. The number of such facilities has swollen to more than a thousand.

- *Other public programs.* Heritage Day Health Centers, in Columbus, Ohio, operates a program for adults in the same building as a child-care center sponsored by the YWCA. Both sponsors pool their resources and promote activities including finger painting, cooking, and volleyball. In Lexington, Kentucky, senior centers have been established inside the walls at three high schools, one elementary school, and one middle school. The seniors and students have their own space but share the cafeteria, restrooms, and gymnasium.

    These kinds of programs ensure that the mature and the young are exposed to one another in a positive way. A Johns Hopkins University study found that adults who volunteered in the Baltimore public schools reported increased physical strength. Another study observed forty-eight adult volunteers over the course of a week at a shared site and found that the adults who interacted with children exhibited clear improvement in their disposition.

    A study that looked at two hundred preschoolers in Ohio compared the social skills of those in a shared facility with those in regular day care. The shared-site toddlers scored higher in social development, especially in manners (such as saying "please" and "thank you"). To learn more about intergenerational volunteer opportunities go to the Generations United Web site; it has links to many great programs, such as one at Penn State, which sponsors programs that unite old and young volunteers for environmental education, community planning, farming, child care, and child tutoring.

- *Religious organizations.* Religious groups and institutions can play a great role in harnessing the capabilities of mature adults and in helping to reweave the generational fabric. We are particularly impressed with the way the Church of Jesus Christ of Latter-Day Saints views this dynamic. As Ken has learned through his friendship with North Castle (www.NorthCastlePartners.com) business partner Brent Knudsen, Mormons place an enormous amount of value on family relationships and believe that everyone should give a part of themselves to those less fortunate throughout their lives. In addition, the practice of young men and women serving on missions in faraway places more fully ingrains the importance of selfless giving. We are impressed with how the Mormon Church has already begun to envision a new role for society's elders. In a recent speech by Boyd Packer, acting president of the Quorum of the Twelve Apostles, Packer challenged his congregation by stating, "In your golden years, there is so much to do and so much to be. Do not withdraw into a retirement from life, into amusement. That, for some, would be useless, even selfish." The LDS Church is actively instituting a wide range of new roles and activities for elders interested in helping others in their own communities and throughout the world. These include volunteer missions where older adults are able to use the skills they've developed in areas such as medicine and engineering in less developed countries, managing food storage and genealogy centers, and supporting local church leaders in the affairs of local congregations.

These programs and others like them are just a start. No organization has yet built the visibility that will galvanize our generation, show us all the possibilities, make us feel a part of something bigger, and light our way for the unprecedented era of volunteerism to unfold.

The biggest obstacle to adult volunteerism, it turns out, is that mature folks report that they don't know where to go for information. Eighty-four percent of retirees say they would volunteer if asked. What might they do? GO SERV studied the issue for California and found that among adults ready to volunteer, 39 percent wanted to read with children, 32 percent wanted to teach or tutor, and 30 percent wanted to mentor children. Notice the common thread. Retirees crave interaction with young people. That's encouraging because there's never been a more important time for the generations to connect and understand one another. This is where volunteer opportunities can truly bridge the growing generational divide.

Margaret Mead said, "Somehow we have to get older people back close to growing children if we are to restore a sense of community, a knowledge of the past, and a sense of the future." Mead understood that intergenerational ties cut both ways. Laura Pulford, fourteen, of Montello, Wisconsin, lost her grandparents early in life. Seeking to fill that void, she joined Teenpower, a local youth-led community service organization. She began visiting the nearby Hometown Village apartments every other week, and there she met Ernie Vohland, eighty-five, who astounded her with stories of when he was a milkman delivering dairy products each day by horse-drawn wagon. Ernie evolved into a surrogate grandfather. Laura relishes his first-hand history lessons and says "going to Hometown Village has helped me see how nice and sweet older people are." As for Ernie, he says "that so-called gap you read about, it isn't there. We're not so darn far apart."

Such interaction not only helps keep adults alive and active and relevant, it also keeps the kids open to older folks. Kids can grow up exposed to the aging process and see it as natural, and they can develop a tendency to want to help that will serve them for a lifetime.

Giving Back Is Food for the Soul

Finding the right volunteer activity may take a bit of effort, no question. But giving of yourself to something meaningful simply makes for a better life. As you enter your power years the range and depth of volunteer possibilities will multiply.

Volunteering is a way for you to:

Make a difference. When you ask for nothing in return, you are free to pursue exactly what makes you feel best. According to LaFrance Associates, 77 percent of adult volunteers give their time because doing so makes them feel like they have accomplished something. They made a difference in someone's life.

Kincey Potter, sixty-three, of Annapolis, Maryland, was in the World Trade Center on September 11, 2001. She emerged from the wreckage without injury and with a new appreciation for life. "I had been working very hard, traveling four days a week," says Potter, who for twenty years was a technology project manager who installed the systems Royal Bank of Canada needed to get into online banking. "I thought to myself that life is just too short. I wanted to get to know my neighbors and hometown. I wanted to be part of my community."

For a while she dabbled in real estate, buying homes and fixing them up for sale. But that didn't satisfy her yen to get involved and do something good for her community, so she began volunteering one day a week at the South River Federation, a civic group whose mission was to clean up the heavily polluted South River in her hometown. She was instantly struck by how much this group was able to accomplish. "At work parties, we'd move rocks and spread sand and plant shrubs and grass," she says. "When I saw all of this I thought, wow, this group really does something. They don't just have meetings."

Potter was so moved that she stepped up her pace of activity and became the group's president. She's used her business skills and knowledge of software to modernize the organization's fund-raising efforts, recruit more members, and expand its influence; she's even added two full-time paid positions so the group can be more proactive and efficient. She devotes thirty-five hours a week to the group—and she is not in one of the paid positions. "As I've grown older I have come to realize that, for example, the Chesapeake Bay has almost died in my lifetime. We are not leaving the legacy for our children that we had when we came into the world. Because of human encroachment, we're doing things to the air and water that if we're not careful we will never be able to recover from. This is my way to try to reverse that."

Potter's group has had many successes, including halting a housing development on the river long enough to force the builder to take steps to avoid further polluting the water. "This something I'm passionate about it," Potter says. "It allows me to do something beneficial for the community, and I find that all the skills I developed in twenty years in business are coming in very handy. It's wonderful to be able to use those skills for a cause I think is worthwhile."

Leave a legacy. Everyone would like to be remembered for something; 74 percent in the LaFrance survey said they would volunteer as long as the opportunity was meaningful. They wanted others to remember them for having done something good. In the classic movie *Zorba the Greek*, there is an emotional scene in which a sickly woman lies dying in a room in a traditional Greek village. Surrounding her home and awaiting her final breath are dozens of the village's older women, all dressed in black head veils. When she dies in Zorba's arms, the villagers immediately pour into her home, taking everything. Since this woman had no spouse, children, or preconsidered legacy to leave, within moments of her death, nothing remained of her life. Surely none of us wants to die this way.

Bev Pavlick, fifty-nine, of Warren, New Jersey, was a human resources manager at AT&T for thirty-one years before retiring. Over the next few years she volunteered in the AT&T Pioneers, a group of former and current employees in the telecommunication industry that raises money for charitable causes. But she longed for a more direct way to make a difference. She found it quite accidentally when a fellow alum of her alma mater, St. Francis University, asked if she would consider representing the university at college fairs in the Northeast. "I thought, hmmm, I could do that. My HR skills are transferable to that kind of thing. I didn't need the job, which paid $25,000 a year. But I was getting a little restless and thought this would be a fun way to make a contribution to my old school. I wanted to help. I received a wonderful education there and felt passionate about giving something back."

The importance of creating and leaving a legacy has deep roots. Stephen Sapp, Ph.D., professor of religious studies at the University of Miami, calls attention to the old-fashioned practice of composing an "ethical will," which goes far beyond the transfer of money and property. Sapp explains the immeasurable value of people expressing "the wisdom they have gained during their lifetimes . . . their insights into what makes for a good and fulfilling life, bequeathing a spiritual legacy that may not only outlive whatever material goods they pass on but be of even more real value." Sapp reflects that although the idea of ethical wills was introduced within Jewish traditions during biblical times, we might all do well to consider both the material and nonmaterial legacies we might build and pass on.

Feel more alive. Adults who volunteer live longer, studies have shown, a finding that prompts Harvard political scientist Robert Putnam to declare that civic engagement is the health club of the twenty-first century. A thirteen-year study by Harvard's School of Public Health found that social connection, often achieved through volunteerism, is more important than diet or exercise for health in later life.

Ken tells this story of an exchange that took place with his Grandfather Max years ago:

> My mother's dad, Max Siderman, was a wonderful and kindhearted man who spent his life fixing cars. When I was young, I didn't think this was much of a big deal until I learned that as a very young man in the early years of the twentieth century, he had owned the very first car in his hometown of Newark, New Jersey, and that he was considered the most gifted automobile technician in the area. As a teenager, I would often spend time with him in his magical workshop situated in his rundown garage in which he would gather his tools and his imagination and build the most incredible things. I'd watch as he would cause lamps, toys, and all manner of furniture and gadgets to spring to life. It wasn't quite Giuseppe's workshop—but to me it was close.
>
> A few years later, my grandfather was beaten down by a series of heart attacks and because of his weakened state he could no longer work the heavy tools and equip-

ment in his garage. So in his retirement, he taught himself to sew. And he became really good at it. He started out by fixing the hems on his daughters' and grandaughters' skirts, and then he began to experiment with fabric collages and wall hangings.

Then, as his health continued to decline, he became intensely immersed in a secret sewing project. By then I was away at college but came home regularly to see my friends, brother, parents, and grandparents. We all knew that my grandfather was doing something with the odd assortment of fabric samples my Aunt Marion was bringing to him and that it was taking up much of his time— but he wouldn't let any of the ten grandchildren know exactly what he was doing.

Then one day when I was in my early twenties, my grandmother called me and explained that my grandfather had a gift for me. On my next trip east, after the usual hugs and kisses, my grandfather reached behind a table and pulled out an eight-sided wall hanging made of odd fabrics that had been stitched together, with his favorite photo of me in the center. Over the picture he wrote: "Your Future Is in the Stars." I still cherish this gift, which is on the wall before me now as I write this passage. He had taken weeks to create something I could remember him by. I also learned that he was hard at work creating similar wall hangings for my brother Alan and his other eight grandchildren. Not long after finishing, he passed away.

I believe that my grandfather had realized he was nearing the end of his life, and having no material wealth to pass to us he instead stitched a part of himself into the creation of something—a legacy—that would live on forever. What are you stitching together for the next generation?

The Big Challenge of the Power Years

Okay, so we've made the case that in your power years you'll have more time for fun, friends, family, learning, and anything else that rings your bell. We've shown you ways to fund these dreams and pleasures. Here's the catch: you'll have to decide if you'll gear all of this free time and capacity to self-indulgence—or whether you've got the spirit to take some portion of yourself and your future and share it with others.

Will you be up to the task of playing your part to help improve our world? We hope so. Our generation's longer and healthier life, our unprecedented level of talent, and our drive to stay in the game years longer set the stage for a transformational revolution in which we can marshal our talents and resources and put them to good like no generation before us.

Although we were branded the "youth generation," it may turn out that our brightest period is our maturity.

We're not asking that you give up all the fun and pleasures you're anticipating, but rather that you take some part of you and do something good for others with it. This doesn't have to be a high-pressure assignment. Volunteering an hour a month is better than nothing at all—but an hour a week might be even more satisfying. And you don't have to follow the pack; you can pick and choose whatever you'd feel good doing.

In addition to providing speaking and consulting pro bono for various not-for-profit organizations as well as contributing a good deal of time and financial resources to the nonprofit Esalen Institute (www.Esalen.org)—where his interest in the human potential movement took root—Ken wants to volunteer at his area high school tutoring kids on public speaking. This past year, Ken's daughter Casey leads the volunteering charge for the Dychtwald family through her efforts at a nearby soup kitchen for the homeless. Dan is planning volunteer coaching and leading writing classes. His teenage daughter, Lexie, volunteers teaching English to Hispanics at a nearby community center. Dan's teen son, Kyle, comes home beaming each week after his time volunteering as a teacher's aide for second graders in religious education. Dan's wife, Kim, plans to spend her power years studying and improving the lives of the homeless.

What will be your mission and your legacy? Will you make a mark, or will you fade into a meaningless "Gerassic Park" of unending play and self-absorption? Will you leave the planet having taken more than you have given? Will you use the gift of longevity to obsess about your wrinkles, or to rise to your greatest height?

What organization would be lucky to have your input and guidance? What community activity could benefit from a few hours of your time? Which up-and-coming entrepreneur could be helped by your knowledge and experience? What kind of contribution would make you feel great? Ultimately, how do you want to be remembered at the end of your days?

As a generation we have had the wind at our backs for a lifetime. Our immense numbers have decreed that for economic reasons everyone else organizes his or her affairs around us. Perhaps it's our turn to do something for everyone else. To do so we must transform the current late-life model of withdrawal and entitlement into a new paradigm. We need to gather our lifetime of learning and experience and our generation's extensive talents and give back our time and money to attack poverty, illiteracy, oppression, crime, and the many other ills that detract from daily life and diminish the future for our children and their children.

We've been blessed. We have changed the world. Now we must change the system one more time, setting a path toward a maturity that is not a vast period of retreat and decline but one of remarkable contribution. We believe that therein lies your and our destiny—a true legacy.

We will either be remembered as history's largest generation or its greatest. The choice is ours.

Authors' Note

As your power years unfold, we'd like to hear how you're doing. Please e-mail us your account of any bold and exciting turning points in your life. We'd like to know why you made the decisions you made and how it all worked out, and of any regrets or reflections on the opportunities you may have missed.

One key moment we're acutely interested in: when the kids leave home and you become an empty nester. Are you doing anything unusual to stay in touch with them? How have you managed your sense of loss? How are you spending all that sudden extra time and money—beyond warm-weather travel and simple leisure pursuits? Have you grown closer to your spouse or further apart? What are you doing about it? What surprises does this period hold for you, and how are you responding?

Please tell us about your fun new job or philanthropic calling. We'd like to know how you're navigating the power years dating scene. Have you discovered any unusual leisure, employment, or other opportunities? What new or unusual living arrangements are you trying? Anything special about the way you started your power-years small business? Any concerns or issues that we've missed?

You get the idea. We're looking for illustrative and poignant stories to help us document this emerging period of life. If you have a tale, please tell it in an e-mail (be as brief as possible) to poweryearsstories@agewave.com. Kindly include your full name, day and night phone numbers, and your address. We'll read every word, but cannot promise a response. Thank you for your attention, and best of luck with the rest of your life.

Sincerely,

Ken Dychtwald
Dan Kadlec

Notes

Unless otherwise noted, all passages are paraphrased except for sections in direct quotes:

Chapter 2: New Ways to Have Fun

31   *"Empty-nesters are really prime"*   St. Paul Pioneer Press, August 28, 2004.

32   *After John Tronco married*   Business Journal, Charlotte, North Carolina, March 1, 2004.

33   *Curt and Jeanne Schryer looked forward to the day*   Kiplinger's magazine, March 2003.

37   *When they were young*   Express, January 9, 2003.

38   *For Erma Marak, new adventures helped*   recordnet.com, November 5, 2002.

38   *Travel adventure helped Carol Madsen*   Boston Globe, July 28, 2002

40   *Phil Hendrix, a retired teacher*   recordnet.com, November 5, 2002.

41   *Garth Fisher tackled the Applachian trail*   Trailjournals.com.

44   *Dorothy Robinson of Stockton, California, travels*   recordnet.com, November 5, 2002.

46   *Seeking to expand her horizons, Shige Kanei*   The Asahi Shimbun, April 2, 2002.

46   *Allen Young had always admired*   ecochallengeat.com testimonials.

Chapter 3: Rediscovering and Forging Vital Relationships

51 *New Yorkers Debra and Gary Kreissman* *Wall Street Journal*, March 3, 2000.

56 *Different couples honor and rediscover* *Arizona Republic*, February 12, 2003.

65 *happened with Carl and Mary Ann* *AARP*, September and October 2003.

69 *Jan grew depressed after* *Arizona Republic*, May 2, 2003.

72 *A few years ago, the noted* *AARP*, March and April 2004.

74 *Only one in three of today's* *St. Paul Pioneer Press*, February 3, 2004.

75 *A simple Christmas tradition* Generation United Testimonials.

76 *Many camps now cater* *Time*, July 21, 2003.

77 *William and Lillian Luby were determined* *Chicago Tribune*, December 13, 2003.

Chapter 4: Creating Your New Dream Job

83 *After thirty-seven years as a marketing* *Time*, July 20, 2002.

88 *Joan Schweighardt did it* 2young2retire.com.

89 *Workplace connections are what drive* *USA Today*, September 1, 2000.

89 *Brian Naber was the president* *Ohio*, June 1, 2002.

90 *Opthalmologist Herve M. Bryon* 2young2retire.com.

93 *Charles Romeo, the head of human resources* *Chicago Tribune*, June 16, 1997.

94 *"What we don't want to see happen"* *Business Insurance*, April 8, 2002.

98 *For twenty years Tim Tingle* 2young2retire.com.

99 *When she was growing up, Helena Hale* helenahale.com.

101 *George Rogers, retired after thirty years* *American Demographics*, November 30, 2000.

105 *At Aerospace Corporation* *HRMagazine*, December 1, 2001.

106 *"We introduced phased retirement"* *Chicago Tribune*, June 11, 2000.

109 *Anne Kleine, a career nurse* score.org.

Chapter 5: Lifelong Learning Adventures

120 *Michael Olmstead, pastor* Springfield (MO) News-Leader, January 17, 2004.

121 *Being a beginner in adulthood* Chicago Daily Herald, May 17, 2002.

126 *Charlotte and Harold Feldman* Harvard-magazine.com.

128 *June Sims of Ada, Oklahoma* New Choices, December 2000/January 2001.

135 *"The intellectual aspect of the organization"* St. Petersburg Times, June 18, 1997.

136 *That's the way Clint Stirling* University of Phoenix Web site.

138 *World Explorer cruises ripped out* vancourier.com.

139 *The food is great* nichedirectories.com.

139 *Richard, a retired math professor* adulted.about.com.

Chapter 6: Where and How to Live

150 *There are people such as Dr. Robert Conn* Time files by Leslie Whitaker, February 2002.

153 *For twenty-one years, the two-story* St. Paul Pioneer Press, August 28, 2004.

154 *While some people seek to downsize* Crain's Detroit Business, September 6, 2004.

154 *Some people will seek to live* Better Homes and Gardens, July 2003.

166 *John and Betty Jean Rife found* Associated Press, April 2004.

166 *After more than twenty years of living* Kiplinger's, November 2002.

Chapter 8: Leaving a Legacy

215 *Jean Jones found new meaning* Generations United testimonials.

224 *When he retired, Frank Leibold* Fast Company, September 2004.

228 *Laura Pulford, fourteen, of Montello* Generations United testimonials.

Index